ROSEMARY CONLEY

Rosemary Conley is Britain's most successful diet and fitness guru, with 25 years' experience of helping people to lose weight and get fitter. It was in 1986, as a result of a gall bladder problem, that she started to follow a low-fat diet in an attempt to avoid surgery. She discovered that this way of eating stream-lined her body in a way she'd never been able to achieve on previous diets. Keen to share this knowledge with others, she decided to put her experiences on paper. The result was her *Hip and Thigh Diet*, which was published in 1988 and captured the imagination of the nation. This book and its sequel, *Rosemary Conley's Complete Hip and Thigh Diet*, have dominated the best-seller lists for eight years and have sold in excess of two million copies.

Subsequent books and videos have all been instant bestsellers, and Rose-mary's realistic and achievable diet and fitness programmes have brought hope and motivation to millions of women who have successfully slimmed down and toned up the Conley way. Total book and video sales exceed four million and two million respectively. When asked why her products have been so successful in such a highly competitive marketplace, Rosemary says: 'It's because my diets and exercises work, and they work for ordinary, real people.'

In 1993 the Rosemary Conley Diet & Fitness Clubs were launched across the United Kingdom, fulfilling a need to give additional support to followers of Rosemary's diets in a positive and welcoming environment. Operating under a franchise system, carefully selected instructors are fully trained to teach the Rosemary Conley philosophy. It is the fastest growing franchise operation in the United Kingdom, with 175 franchisees currently running over 2,000 classes throughout the country and 60,000 members coming through their doors each week. It is the first national diet and fitness organ-isation where only qualified instructors are in operation. In 1995 the com-pany received the British Franchise Association's Newcomer of the Year Award.

January 1996 saw the launch of the exciting new Rosemary Conley Diet & Fitness Magazine. With contributions from leading experts in the fields of nutrition, health and fitness, it is one of the most authoritative magazines in its field.

In 1996 Rosemary was appointed a consultant to Marks & Spencer, to help them develop their Healthy Choice range of food.

Rosemary maintains a high media profile with regular television and radio appearances. She is diet and fitness expert on Granada's popular *This Morn-ing* programme, and since October 1996 she has hosted her own pro-gramme, *Diet and Fitness with R* on GSB's Health and Beauty c'

Rosemary lives in mington, with whom she runs ley Diet & Fitness Clubs Limit a daugh-ter by her first marriag

D1464395

ALSO IN ARROW BY ROSEMARY CONLEY

Rosemary Conley's Hip and Thigh Diet

Rosemary Conley's Complete Hip and Thigh Diet

Rosemary Conley's Inch Loss Plan

*Rosemary Conley's Hip and
Thigh Diet Cookbook* (with Patricia Bourne)

Rosemary Conley's Metabolism Booster Diet

Rosemary's Whole Body Programme
(published jointly with the BBC)

*Rosemary Conley's New Hip and
Thigh Diet Cookbook* (with Patricia Bourne)

Shape Up For Summer

Rosemary Conley's Beach Body Plan

Rosemary Conley's Flat Stomach Plan

Be Slim! Be Fit!

Rosemary Conley's Complete Flat Stomach Plan

Rosemary Conley's

NEW BODY PLAN

ARROW

Published by Arrow Books in 1997

1 3 5 7 9 10 8 6 4 2

© Rosemary Conley Enterprises 1997

The right of Rosemary Conley to be identified as the author of this work has been asserted by her in accordance with the Copyright, Designs and Patents Act, 1988

Arrow Books Limited
20 Vauxhall Bridge Road, London SW1V 2SA

Random House, Australia (Pty) Limited
16 Dalmore Drive, Scoresby,
Victoria 3179, Australia

Random House New Zealand Limited
18 Poland Road, Glenfield,
Auckland 10, New Zealand

Random House, South Africa (Pty) Limited
Endulini, 5a Jubilee Road, Parktown 2193, South Africa

Random House UK Limited Reg. No. 954009

A CIP catalogue record for this book is available
from the British Library

Papers used by Random House UK Limited are natural, recyclable products made from wood grown in sustainable forests. The manufacturing processes conform to the environmental regulations of the country of origin

ISBN 0 09 918542 3

Printed and bound in Great Britain by
Cox & Wyman, Reading, Berks

IMPORTANT

If you have a medical condition or are pregnant, the diet and exercises described in this book should not be followed without first consulting your doctor. All guidelines and warnings should be read carefully, and the author and publisher cannot accept responsibility for injuries or damage arising out of a failure to comply with the same.

Contents

This healthy eating and fitness programme is in keeping with current nutritional guidelines and is suitable for anyone who is seeking to make long-term changes to their eating and exercise habits. The calorie allowance is set at the optimum level for successful weight loss and, certainly, the option to have between-meal snacks can be effective in helping the slimmer to adhere to the diet. Low-fat eating combined with regular exercise is the best formula for a healthy lifestyle and is particularly important for weight maintenance. This book puts that message across in an easy-to-follow and positive way.

Dr Andrew Prentice, MRC Dunn
Clinical Nutrition Centre, Cambridge

Anyone who is overweight and who follows the advice in this book will reduce their body weight and size. To maintain these benefits, the principles described need to be followed in the long term. Failure to do so may result in your regaining your lost weight.

From your interest in this book it is clear that you either have an interest in health, or it is possible that you have an underlying problem with your eating habits. In extreme cases, this could manifest itself as an eating disorder which requires more help than this book can offer. In this instance, I would encourage you to seek further help via your GP or other nutritional specialist, or contact the Eating Disorders Association on 01603 621414.

Acknowledgements

With each book that I write I become acutely aware of the great team who surround me and enable me to achieve an end result which I hope will be greatly enjoyed by many. This book is no exception and, as I have become increasingly busy over the last year, the contribution made by my team is appreciated more than ever.

Researching the latest products on the market for inclusion in the diet is a mammoth task in itself and I must thank Linda Stevens and Julia Martin for their endless trips to the supermarkets on my behalf.

The exercise section is a crucial part of this book and I want to thank Mary Morris for her expertise and direction in coming up with the most effective workout ever. Mary's support and encouragement knows no bounds, and I am so grateful to her for that. Thank you also to Sue Marcantonio James for her valuable contribution to the exercise section. With such experts around me I know my readers are given the best possible help and guidance.

Thanks must also go to my PA, Louise Cowell, and my assistant, Melody Patterson, who have worked tirelessly in transcribing the many tapes of dictation and the numerous recipes that were so kindly contributed by members of Rosemary Conley Diet & Fitness Clubs.

Special thanks must also go to Patricia Bourne for testing and adapting the recipes in this book to ensure that you get perfect results each time you prepare them.

Any book that is written has to be edited so that it can be read logically and easily. Jan Bowmer has edited my books for many years. Not only does she work incredibly hard on my behalf, she is extremely good at what she does. Jan, I can't thank you enough for sorting out my batches of manuscript and making them into a readable book.

Thanks must also go to the designer, Roger Walker, and the art director, Dennis Barker. You always do such a great job.

Thank you all very much indeed.

1

What's New about the New Body Plan?

Would you like to wear a size 10 or 12 dress that fitted all over? Are you happy with parts of your body but wish that the bigger bits were more in proportion with the smaller ones? I know what it's like – I've been there! For years I hated my lower half, but once I discovered the incredible benefits of low-fat eating, my previously outsized hips and thighs reduced to a 'normal' size and everything became in proportion. That was 10 years ago and since then I've researched and developed that simple dieting principle. The result is a finely tuned weight-loss programme of diet and fitness, as described in this book, that gives incredible results very, very easily.

That's why I believe my New Body Plan is the most effective diet and fitness programme ever. It combines six meals a day, which will prevent those hunger pangs and avoid wholesale bingeing, with a very effective form of exercising called New Body.

In my previous diets I have recommended that slimmers eat three meals a day and avoid the habit of snacking in between meals, as I feel strongly that anyone who wants to lose weight should educate themselves towards set mealtimes when they eat plenty and feel satisfied. It is very important that the slimmer does not feel deprived, and having a substantial meal three times a day helps to build confidence in their eating patterns and has proved effective in minimising binge eating.

However, many slimmers have asked me for a diet that will allow them to eat something between meals since, because of their lifestyles, they find themselves really hungry at certain times. These weak moments tend to occur at three key points in the day: late in the morning (if they eat an early breakfast), in the afternoon at children's teatime and at around 9pm (if they eat their evening meal at, say, 6pm). Late-night nibbling can often lead to a wholesale binge, but with a regular pattern of six meals a day, as offered in this New Body Plan, bingeing should become a thing of the past.

The calorie content of this diet is around 1400 calories a day for women. Men can increase the quantities by 25 per cent or, if they are a manual worker, by 50 per cent. All menus and snacks are low in fat, but sufficient fat is included within the diet to ensure optimum nutrition. Care has been taken to include plenty of foods that are rich in calcium and iron and, providing that you eat a varied diet from the menus suggested, you should be obtaining sufficient nutrients.

The rate of weight loss you can expect on this plan will vary between individuals. The more overweight you are, the more weight you will lose initially. But the maximum weight loss will be achieved by those who stick rigidly to the diet plan and who exercise regularly.

New Body is the name given to a unique exercise system designed to reshape the body. It's a safe and incredibly effective workout which combines low-impact aerobic moves with controlled body conditioning exercises that strengthen and tone the muscles. The result is a honed down and toned up body – the kind of body you would never believe could be yours.

Aerobic exercise – that's any exercise which makes you puff – strengthens the heart and lungs and burns fat, while *toning* exercises work specific muscle groups to strengthen and tone the body and improve our overall shape. My New Body Workout combines both these elements, thus enabling you to work out in an effective and time-efficient way. The workout is divided into six sections, each of which focuses on a specific area of the body so that you can design your own workout and concentrate on your particular problem area.

Try to do the exercises at least three times a week, but if you do them on six days out of seven, you'll see the fastest results. If you have a video player at home, you may like to try my New Body By Design video where I work out with two successful slimmers and show different variations on different moves (see back of book for details).

Think about general activity in your everyday life, too. The more physically active you are at any time of the day, the more calories you will burn, the more fat you will lose and the slimmer you will become. Try not to think of your diet and fitness campaign as something you do for half an hour a day and at meal-times. It should be a new lifestyle which becomes a habit that will bring you abounding energy and a new zest for life.

I don't doubt that at some point during the next few weeks you will find yourself tempted away from the guidelines of the New Body Plan. You're only human, after all. To help you cope with these difficult times I have included a special Willpower Booster Plan in Chapter 8. At those times when you feel depleted of willpower, please turn to this chapter to find some inspiration to keep you on the straight and narrow. But remember, nothing tastes as good as being slim feels!

2
Dispelling the Metabolism Myths

Many people who fail to lose weight blame their lack of success on their metabolism. They believe that theirs is slower than most people's and that they only need to look at a cream cake to gain a couple of pounds. In reality the metabolic rate – the rate at which we burn calories – does vary from one person to another, but, interestingly, if you are overweight, then your metabolic rate is actually likely to be higher, not lower, than that of a slimmer person.

Obesity expert Dr Andrew Prentice, who is based at the Dunn Clinical Nutrition Centre in Cambridge, has been involved in numerous clinical studies on metabolism. At the Dunn Centre they have special sealed units called metabolic chambers where people come and stay for up to 14 days at a time to participate in controlled experiments. These chambers are like bed-sitting rooms and are comfortably furnished with a bed, washbasin, toilet facilities, table, chair, stereo, video and an exercise bike. Each room is completely airtight with a special seal around the door. A two-way hatch facilitates the serving of carefully calculated meals and the removal of waste products in the appropriate receptacles! The air within each unit is circulated throughout a special ventilated system. This allows the oxygen breathed in and the carbon dioxide produced by the person inside to be measured accurately. These measurements are then used to calculate exactly how much energy (calories) per minute is being used up. A computer printout running constantly shows any increase or decrease in activity and the appropriate fluctuation in energy output.

I paid a visit to the Dunn Nutrition Centre while I was recording a series of films for Granada's *This Morning* programme. We wanted to demonstrate scientifically the difference in the metabolic rate of two people who had different body weights. A member of one of our classes in Norfolk had successfully lost six stone but had since reached a plateau and felt frustrated that she was apparently unable to shift her final few stones to reach her target weight. Gail was the perfect candidate, having reduced from 22 stone to 16 stone, but she believed her metabolic rate was the reason her weight was sticking. She felt her metabolic rate had slowed down to around 300 calories a day. It was agreed that I would be the other candidate on the basis that many people would assume that I had a high metabolic rate in view of the regular exercise I take and the fact that I'm not overweight.

So Gail and I were placed in a metabolic chamber for around 24 hours. Then we were instructed to lie on the bed absolutely motionless for one hour. During this time a very careful and accurate reading was taken of our respective metabolic rates. At the end of the session we were allowed to get up, wash, dress and emerge from our quarters to wait for the results to be announced. The computer provided the proof that my basal metabolic rate (BMR) was 1343. This was the number of calories I needed to fuel my body throughout the day without even getting out of bed. As soon as I became active, obviously the number of calories burned would increase.

Gail's BMR was no less than 1900 calories! This was significantly higher than mine and was due to the fact that she was a larger lady – in fact, she weighed twice as much as I did. Gail was amazed, and even more so when Doctor Prentice told her that as soon as she became active in her normal daily life she would be burning up another 800–900 calories, making a total calorie expenditure of 2700–2800 per day! It is therefore clear to see that if Gail followed a diet of even as much as 1900 calories a day, she would be bound to lose weight. Gail went away feeling very encouraged and was determined to continue with the diet. She realised that previously she must have been eating many more calories than she'd thought.

From this exercise you can see that weight has an important bearing on the basal metabolic rate. If you are carrying some excess weight, then your body requires more calories than that of a slimmer person simply to sustain your existing weight. Age also has a bearing on the BMR. We require less fuel as we get older because our body composition changes somewhat – our muscles tend to become smaller as we tend to be less active. Muscle is an energy-hungry tissue whereas fat is not, therefore, the more muscle we have, the higher the metabolic rate will be. This is why the New Body exercises in this book are so important. Not only will they help you to burn fat, they will also help you to increase your muscle mass (the size of your muscles) and this, in turn, will increase your metabolic rate.

Crash dieting and yo-yo dieting, on the other hand, will have the opposite effect. If you have ever gone on a crash diet or a meal-replacement-type diet or have simply gone without food in the hope that it would effect a swift weight loss, you may have reduced the amount of muscle tissue on your body. This is because, under such starvation conditions, the body starts to burn muscle rather than fat. However, providing you go back to eating sensible, healthy food and sufficient calories to fuel your basal metabolic requirement, and at the same time start doing some specific muscle-toning exercises, you will soon be able to increase your muscle mass and consequently your metabolic rate. It is never too late to start to remedy any damage that might have been done.

We need good, nutritious food to stay healthy. Without it, we may lack energy, age prematurely and be susceptible to a variety of illnesses and infections. The good news is that there are loads of different, healthy, low-fat foods which taste absolutely delicious and leave us feeling more than satisfied, but we need to make them part of our everyday lifestyle.

Now, for the first time, you can estimate your daily calorie requirements by using the metabolic chart on pages 10–12. This will give you an idea of your personal basal metabolic rate (that's the number of calories you need to exist), plus the total number of calories you need to sustain your *existing* weight. To *lose* weight really effectively, you need to eat fewer calories than you expend each day and increase your activity level.

How to use the tables to estimate your daily energy (kilocalorie) needs

First decide how active you are. Take care not to overestimate it. Most people believe they are more active than they really are. Here is a guide:

Sedentary This applies to most people in modern society.
Active To classify as active you must be active at work *or* spend at least two hours per week in a very active leisure pursuit.
Very active To classify as very active you must have a very active occupation (including lifting, carrying and standing for long periods) *or* be extremely active for at least four hours per week in your leisure time – people would describe you as 'very sporty'.

Then select the table appropriate to your age and sex. Read across from your weight to the relevant column. The first column tells you your estimated BMR. The appropriate activity column tells you your total daily energy output. The values are only best estimates and are calculated according to the Department of Health's Dietary Reference Values (1991).

Daily energy (kilocalorie) requirements of women aged 18–29 years

Body weight (stones)	Basal metabolic rate	Total energy requirement (kcal per day)		
		Sedentary	Active	Very active
6	1052	1580	1790	2000
6½	1099	1650	1870	2090
7	1146	1720	1950	2180
7½	1193	1790	2030	2270
8	1240	1860	2110	2360
8½	1288	1930	2190	2450
9	1335	2000	2270	2540
9½	1382	2070	2350	2630
10	1428	2140	2430	2710
10½	1476	2210	2510	2800
11	1523	2880	2590	2890
11½	1570	2360	2670	2980
12	1618	2430	2750	3070
12½	1664	2500	2830	3160
13	1711	2570	2830	3250
13½	1758	2640	2990	3340
14	1806	2710	3070	3430
14½	1853	2780	3150	3520
15	1900	2850	3230	3610

Daily energy (kilocalorie) requirements of women aged 30–59 years

Body weight (stones)	Basal metabolic rate	Total energy requirement (kcal per day)		
		Sedentary	Active	Very active
6	1163	1740	1980	2210
6½	1190	1790	2020	2260
7	1215	1820	2070	2310
7½	1242	1860	2110	2360
8	1268	1900	2160	2410
8½	1295	1940	2200	2460
9	1323	1980	2250	2510
9½	1348	2020	2290	2560
10	1374	2060	2340	2610
10½	1400	2100	2380	2660
11	1427	2140	2430	2710
11½	1454	2180	2470	2760
12	1480	2220	2520	2810
12½	1505	2260	2560	2860
13	1532	2300	2600	2910
13½	1559	2340	2650	2960
14	1586	2380	2700	3010
14½	1612	2420	2740	3060
15	1639	2460	2790	3110

Daily energy (kilocalorie) requirements of women aged 60 years and over

Body weight (stones)	Basal metabolic rate	Total energy requirement (kcal per day)		
		Sedentary	Active	Very active
6	940	1410	1600	1790
6½	970	1460	1650	1840
7	998	1500	1700	1900
7½	1028	1542	1750	1950
8	1057	1590	1800	2010
8½	1087	1630	1850	2070
9	1116	1670	1900	2120
9½	1146	1720	1950	2180
10	1174	1760	2000	2230
10½	1204	1810	2050	2290
11	1233	1850	2100	2340
11½	1263	1890	2150	2400
12	1292	1940	2200	2450
12½	1320	1980	2240	2510
13	1350	2030	2300	2570
13½	1380	2070	2350	2620
14	1409	2110	2400	2680
14½	1439	2160	2450	2730
15	1469	2200	2500	2790

Daily energy (kilocalorie) requirements of men aged 18–29 years

Body weight (stones)	Basal metabolic rate	Total energy requirement (kcal per day)		
		Sedentary	Active	Very active
8	1456	2180	2480	2770
8½	1509	2260	2570	2870
9	1557	2340	2650	2960
9½	1606	2410	2730	3050
10	1652	2480	2810	3140
10½	1701	2550	2890	3230
11	1749	2620	2970	3320
11½	1797	2700	3060	3410
12	1846	2770	3140	3510
12½	1892	2840	3220	3600
13	1940	2910	3300	3690
13½	1990	2980	3380	3780
14	2037	3060	3460	3870
14½	2086	3130	3550	3960
15	2134	3200	3630	4050
15½	2180	3270	3710	4140
16	2220	3330	3770	4220
16½	2278	3420	3870	4330
17	2330	3490	3950	4420

Daily energy (kilocalorie) requirements of men aged 30–59 years

Body weight (stones)	Basal metabolic rate	Total energy requirement (kcal per day)		
		Sedentary	Active	Very active
8	1458	2190	2480	2770
8½	1495	2240	2540	2840
9	1532	2300	2600	2910
9½	1569	2350	2670	2980
10	1604	2410	2730	3050
10½	1641	2460	2790	3120
11	1678	2520	2850	3190
11½	1715	2570	2920	3260
12	1752	2630	2980	3330
12½	1787	2680	3040	3400
13	1824	2740	3100	3470
13½	1861	2790	3160	3540
14	1898	2850	3230	3640
14½	1934	2900	3290	3680
15	1970	2960	3350	3750
15½	2007	3010	3410	3810
16	2037	3060	3460	3870
16½	2080	3120	3540	3950
17	2117	3180	3600	4020

Daily energy (kilocalorie) requirements of men aged 60 years and over

Body weight (stones)	Basal metabolic rate	Total energy requirement (kcal per day)		
		Sedentary	Active	Very active
8	1306	1960	2220	2480
8½	1344	2020	2280	2550
9	1382	2070	2350	2630
9½	1420	2130	2410	2700
10	1457	2190	2480	2770
10½	1494	2240	2540	2840
11	1533	2300	2610	2910
11½	1571	2360	2670	2980
12	1609	2410	2740	3060
12½	1646	2470	2800	3130
13	1684	2530	2860	3200
13½	1722	2580	2930	3270
14	1760	2640	2990	3340
14½	1798	2700	3060	3420
15	1836	2750	3120	3490
15½	1873	2810	3180	3560
16	1904	2860	3240	3620
16½	1949	2920	3310	3700
17	1988	2980	3380	3780

Prepared by Dr Andrew Prentice, MRC Dunn Clinical Nutrition Centre, Cambridge

How to speed up your metabolism

Eating regular meals will ensure that the body receives a steady supply of nutrients that can be utilised to provide energy as well as growth and repair. During the day the body's energy systems take a leading role, enabling us to carry out our daily activities. At night the energy systems slow down, and the maintenance and repair workers come into action. Any food not processed during the day is sorted and fully digested while we are asleep, and the various nutrients are taken around the body and deposited where they are needed. Any waste matter is then left in our waste products' department, ready for elimination in the morning. When we wake up after a good night's sleep we are delighted to find a flat stomach, which represents an empty fuel tank awaiting a delivery of energy at breakfast time. Breakfast is so important because it kick-starts the metabolism into action, rather like starting an engine.

Over recent years there has been a popular train of thought which suggested that breaking down our daily calorie intake into several, smaller meals a day would increase the metabolic rate. However, in clinical tests no firm evidence was found to support this theory, although there is no doubt that immediately after we have eaten, the metabolic rate does increase for a short period of time. The key, therefore, is to find a way of eating that will effect a steady and healthy weight loss which, at the same time, will satisfy the slimmer to such an extent that they have no inclination to nibble or binge outside of the recommended calorie allowance. It is with this goal in mind that I have written this book. I believe that we are most tempted to cheat at those times of the day when our blood sugar levels fall because of the period of time that has elapsed between meals.

We can increase our metabolic rate by increasing the size of our muscles. We can only do this by making the muscles work harder than normal so that they automatically grow bigger to cope with the extra work we ask them to perform. Muscles are made up of millions of fibres. When we work a muscle we cause it to contract and become bigger. You only need to pick up a 1.8kg (4lb) weight in your hand and bend your arm at the elbow to see your bicep muscle (at the front of the upper arm) become bigger.

If you were to lift that weight several times, you would find that the muscle gradually began to ache. The first time you lifted the weight, perhaps 60 per cent of the fibres in that muscle were called into action. The second time you lifted it, those initial fibres would start to feel a little tired and recruit some more support from another 10–15 per cent of fibres in the muscle. This process would continue with each repetition until eventually the muscle would be using 100 per cent of its pulling power. It now needs to recruit or manufacture some additional fibres to enable it to do the work. This, in turn, makes the muscle bigger and stronger.

This is why when performing strengthening and toning exercises we need to do sufficient repetitions to enable our muscles to be challenged to the point of mild discomfort and then do two more repetitions to ensure that the message is clearly received by the muscles to recruit more fibres. This does not mean that you will end up looking like a weight-lifter – far from it! Weight-lifting is a specialised form of muscle-building which requires the body to use its muscles to the absolute limit. This, in turn, forces the muscles to get bigger and bigger through overuse. In the work-out in this book we will only be working to the point of mild discomfort, which is sufficient to enable the muscles to be challenged but not exhausted.

Toning and strengthening exercises will not only increase the metabolic rate but also improve the health of our bones. Muscles are attached to bones and therefore if the muscles are made to work harder they also stimulate the strength of our bones, encouraging them to become stronger and less brittle. Muscle strengthening and toning exercise is therefore particularly helpful in the prevention of osteoporosis.

There is some evidence that we can further increase the metabolic rate by taking regular aerobic exercise. Aerobic exercise increases the metabolic rate and the benefit continues for some hours after we have finished exercising. This means that if we exercise regularly at a rate that causes us to be slightly out of breath, the metabolic rate will receive a boost.

So to maximise the benefits to your metabolic rate, resolve never to crash diet again. Eat regular meals that are high in nutrition and low in fat to keep your body fat to a minimum. Do strengthening and toning exercises regularly to keep your muscles in good shape. Combine these with an aerobic workout two or three times a week and you will ensure that your metabolic rate is elevated on a regular basis. If you follow my New Body Workout in Chapter 7, you'll receive both toning and aerobic benefits at the same time.

3

The Fat Calorie versus the Carbohydrate Calorie

The energy content of food is measured in kilocalories or kcal for short, also commonly referred to as calories. One gram of fat contains nine calories – that's more than twice the amount of calories contained in carbohydrate or protein, both of which contain around four calories per gram.

When I first devised my Hip and Thigh Diet I proved to myself and to my trial dieters that eating a diet very low in fat was an incredibly effective way of losing unwanted weight and inches. I didn't know why it worked the way it did, I just knew that it did. Since then, scientists have proved that fat calories are much more fattening than carbohydrate calories. This is because the body uses carbohydrate calories in a different way from fat calories.

Scientists at the Dunn Clinical Nutrition Centre have carried out numerous experiments to determine the body's reaction to different types of foods. For the purpose of some of these experiments they used a piece of equipment called a metabolic hood – a kind of ventilated hood. In one study, subjects were given various meals which had been carefully prepared and measured by the staff at the Centre. After each meal was consumed, the hood was placed over the head of each subject. The hood was attached to a machine which measured the amount of oxygen breathed in and the carbon dioxide produced. When the subjects had eaten a high-carbohydrate meal, the machine gave a high reading, illustrating that the body was burning the carbohydrate quickly – rather like turning up the gas on your cooker. A similar reaction was recorded after they had eaten a meal high in protein, say, a lean steak or a meal of chicken. But when the subjects were fed a high-fat meal, say, of chocolate or cheese, the machine hardly registered an increase in energy output.

In other words, carbohydrate foods such as bread, potatoes, rice, cereals and pasta are quickly converted into fuel that is burned easily and rapidly by the body. Protein food is also utilised quickly. However, when you eat fat, it's as if the body doesn't notice that you have consumed it, which proves that fat is ineffective as an instant energy source.

The natural reaction to this information is to think that we can eat carbohydrate and protein freely and the body will just burn it off. Unfortunately it is not quite as simple as that, since if we overeat carbohydrate – or indeed any food – we will store any excess as fat. However, since carbohydrate is burned quickly by the body, this means it is inefficient as a long-term energy store. Fat, on the other hand, is stored very efficiently by the body, which is the opposite of what the slimmer is trying to achieve. Sixty per cent of our daily diet should be in the form of carbohydrate which, in addition to the foods mentioned previously, also includes foods such as fruit and vegetables. Protein, like carbohydrate, is also stored inefficiently by the body, but too much can be harmful, so our intake of protein (foods such as meat, poultry, eggs, fish and cheese) should be kept to moderate levels.

Fat, however, is completely different. Imagine you have fat deposit boxes around the areas of the body where you store most fat. If you are pear-shaped, you'll store most of your fat around your hips and thighs. Apple shapes store fat in the abdomen, and heart shapes are top heavy, with full busts and broad shoulders. Each time you eat fat, imagine that fat is taking a direct route from your mouth to your fat deposit boxes, where it is stored until it is needed by the body to make up any energy deficit.

There are two ways to create an increase in energy requirement and reduce the amount of fat on the body. Firstly, if the number of calories taken in by the body falls below the required level, the body calls on its fat stores to make up the shortfall. Secondly, during moderate aerobic exercise, fat on the body is drawn into the bloodstream and burned as energy in the presence of both oxygen from the air we breathe and glycogen (a chemical found in our muscles), which is created from the carbohydrate we eat.

It is plain to see, therefore, that if we exercise regularly, we will reduce the amount of fat on our bodies, and if at the same time we restrict our fat intake, those fat stores that we have burned away will not be replenished. Consequently, we will become fitter and leaner and, providing that we keep away from high-fat foods in the future, we will stay that way for ever. So remember, next time you are tempted to eat that bar of chocolate or cake oozing with cream, realise that if you eat it you are going to have to wear it!

Does that mean I can eat unlimited amounts of low-fat foods?

Sadly no! All calories count, so even if you eat a very-low-fat diet, if it contains too many calories you will still gain weight in the form of fat. It is just that because the body is inefficient at storing carbohydrate as fat, its inclination is to burn it off, but if you eat carbohydrate in excess, it will almost certainly be stored as fat. Dietary fat, on the other hand is very readily stored.

The key is to restrict your calorie intake to the level of your basal metabolic rate, which on average is around 1400 calories a day for women and 1700 for men. As explained previously, the bigger you are, the higher your basal metabolic rate will be, so a larger than average person will lose weight very efficiently by eating, say, 1800 calories a day. By reducing the fat and at the same time increasing the proportion of carbohydrate in your daily diet, you will be maximising the use of the energy (fuel) you are taking in.

What about those days when I can't help but eat more?

There will always be days when through social engagements or an unplanned business lunch you will end up eating many more calories than you would otherwise choose. Don't use this as an excuse for breaking the diet, but instead try and balance this out by eating a little less later or cutting down the next day. Do not skip any meals, though. Just be extra strict for one day and you will be surprised at how quickly that indulgent meal gets used up by the body. To help things along, try to do more exercise within 24 hours of eating that extra food. This will help you, both physically and psychologically, to get back on to the straight and narrow.

Don't we need a certain amount of fat in the diet?

Yes we do and providing you eat a varied diet you will be eating sufficient fat, since it is found in varying quantities in almost every food that we eat – there is even a trace in lettuce! Fat lurks in all kinds of unlikely places, such as dry bread, lean meat, poultry, egg yolks (the whites are fat-free) cereals, and in a variety of ready-made foods that we buy.

Some fats are more important than others such as the fat found in oily fish. Consequently, oily fish such as salmon, tuna, mackerel and sardines are included in my diet and should be eaten at least once or twice a week, more if you like. Select brands canned in brine.

How many grams of fat should I have on a low-fat diet?

I suggest you never have fewer than 20 and probably not more than 40 grams while you are trying to lose weight. Once you reach your target weight, you can increase your intake up to a maximum of 70 grams a day. However, I recommend that you do not count fat grams, as it is easy to get paranoid about how many we eat in a day, and counting them can become a negative habit. It is far better just to follow the diet plan in this book, which is calculated to fall within these brackets.

When buying any product from the supermarket or food store, always check the nutrition label and select only those products with four grams or less per hundred grams of product. All foods containing four per cent or less fat are acceptable within my diet plan. Of course calories do count, but if you follow the four per cent fat ruling and keep within your daily calorie allowance (approximately 1400 for women and 1700 for men), the fat content will look after itself.

But I thought olive oil was good for you?

All oil, including olive oil, is 100 per cent fat and, while olive oil does have some nutritional qualities, it does not play a part in a weight-reducing low-fat diet except for vegetarians who may be eating less fat than meat-eaters. Vegetarians therefore may include a little oil in their cooking, and extra virgin olive oil is the best choice. The problem with oil is that it looks so harmless and is almost unnoticeable that we don't realise how many fat calories are hidden in that salad tossed in French dressing.

Can I use low-fat spread on my sandwiches?

Many low-fat spreads still have a remarkably high fat content – some contain as much as 60 per cent fat. If you really cannot bear to eat your toast or sandwiches without some form of butter flavoured spread, then you could try Tesco's 95% Fat Free Sunflower Spread, although this is still one per cent over my four per cent ruling. However, I suggest that you try spreading your bread with very-low-fat salad dressing or pickle to add moisture and help prevent any salad filling falling out of the sandwich. It's tasty, too.

Can I have sugar?

Sugar is simple carbohydrate and, while it contains empty calories offering few nutrients, it is an energy-giver. I am not against having a little sugar in moderation. I always have a teaspoon of sugar in my tea and on my cereal. It's my belief that if you have a little sugar in your diet you are less likely to be drawn to confectionery and chocolate, biscuits and cakes, which may be high in fat and are often craved due to a drop in blood sugar levels between meals. The 20 calories contained within a teaspoon of sugar will be burned off within an hour of general activity and will only be stored as fat if taken as part of an excess of calories overall.

Some people suffer quite severe symptoms of feeling dizzy or faint if they go long periods without eating. I have a friend who experienced such symptoms, so I suggested she tried adding sugar to her tea. Since taking this advice, she has noticed a dramatic difference in her energy levels, and all the symptoms have disappeared. It has not adversely affected her weight in any way and she feels 100 per cent better.

What about alcohol?

Alcohol in itself is not the enemy of the dieter, but it does contain calories. Too much alcohol can be harmful to health and therefore it should only be taken in moderation. Accordingly, in my diet I allow one unit of alcoholic drink per day for women and two for men. One unit of alcohol is equivalent to a single measure of spirit, 300ml ($\frac{1}{2}$ pint) of beer or lager, or a glass of wine. If alcohol is taken in excess, it is stored as fat, but a single drink per day will be quickly burned away.

The other big reason for not allowing more alcohol within my diet is that it also affects our willpower. The more alcohol we drink, the more it dilutes our resolve to stick to a diet. Once we become too relaxed, we are more likely to consume far more food than we ought to.

For health reasons, I am unable to exercise, so will I be able to lose weight by dieting alone?

Yes, you can. Obviously exercise would enable you to burn even more calories, but by reducing your fat intake and cutting your calories to around 1300–1400 a day, you should certainly be able to lose weight very efficiently. Don't be disheartened if some weeks your weight stays constant. Perseverance will win the day, but do watch the portion sizes, as we often eat more than we think.

I enjoy exercise but I really don't want to diet. Can I still lose weight?

It is possible to slim down by exercise on its own, but you would need a lot of willpower and quite a lot of time to ensure that you did sufficient exercise for it to be effective in isolation. Running would probably be your most effective way to reduce weight, but you would need to do at least 20 minutes on six days a week. You would also have to take care that you didn't increase your food intake to compensate for the extra energy you would be expending. Low-fat eating isn't like dieting as such, and you may find that simply by adjusting your diet and eating only foods that contain four per cent or less fat you would achieve a satisfactory weight loss.

How fast will I be able to lose weight?

This depends on you and how much weight you have to lose, but it's important to realise that there is a difference between losing weight and losing fat. Losing weight on the scales may give you a high feel-good factor, but it is the inches disappearing that really matters.

If you follow my low-fat diet to the letter, with no cheating, and do the New Body exercises on three to six days a week, you should burn at least 1kg (2lb) of fat off your body per week. Anyone who has a lot of weight to lose may lose more weight than this, but 1kg (2lb) a week is considered a good average. If you think this doesn't sound much, just think that in seven weeks' time you will have lost a stone and be a whole dress size smaller, and that is a big step forward. By eating a reasonable number of calories and by exercising regularly, you will be maximising on your fat loss yet maintaining your muscle mass and increasing your energy levels. Finally, do take the time to measure yourself prior to commencing this diet and exercise programme, as the inch losses will be particularly encouraging.

What happens to all that skin when we lose a lot of weight?

Basically it shrinks, but it shrinks more efficiently if we lose weight gradually by taking regular exercise and eating a low-fat diet. Those who follow crash diets will find that their skin will sag significantly, whereas those who follow a sensible low-fat diet combined with exercise will be pleasantly surprised at how quickly and effortlessly their skin returns to a smaller and quite natural state.

Is it possible to spot reduce?

No. When we follow a weight-reducing, low-fat diet, we tend to lose weight from our fattest areas first.

These areas are often left untouched by weight-reducing diets that don't restrict the dietary fat. As I discovered with my Hip and Thigh Diet, low-fat eating was the only way that I could reduce the fat on my hips and thighs, after endless previous dieting attempts had failed to make any difference to these areas.

4

Getting Your Mind into Gear

When you start a diet you are full of good intentions and your willpower is very strong. You know what you are going to do and you have every belief that this time you will succeed. Depending on your frame of mind and the temptations around you, this determination may hold for several months, or maybe just a few weeks, days or, worse still, only a few hours!

The aim of this chapter is to set out a few suggestions on how you might sustain a good attitude and a positive willpower that will ensure you achieve success. If you anticipate the likely pitfalls and are aware of the danger signals, you will be in a much stronger position to fight back and prevent a downfall.

Stop the bad habits

Habits, whether good ones or bad ones, are easily developed. When we start out on a diet we need to be quite certain that we are going to take steps to curb the bad ones and to consciously develop some good ones.

I have two bad habits which I have to watch carefully. The first is buying soft mints when I buy petrol. I never buy Softmints at any other time, but for some reason when I go into the garage to pay for my petrol I seem to find myself attracted to the little green packets on display. I buy one packet and eat the mints straight off, one after the other, yet if I need to keep a careful watch on my weight because I have a video to record or a photo session looming, I consciously make the decision not to buy any sweets. I then forget all about them and don't even think about buying any for several months – until one day they tempt me again. The next time I go for petrol, I then have the battle of deciding shall I or shall I not buy the mints!

My second temptation is a handful of dry muesli last thing at night as I make a cup of tea before going to bed. Somehow those few minutes before the kettle boils lead me into temptation into the cereal cupboard, and it is the muesli that takes my fancy. I start off with one handful and soon it becomes half a dozen. I am not hungry but temptation strikes. I have to give myself a severe talking to and promise myself that I won't do it again for a week. Soon I forget all about indulging and the habit is broken. So be aware of your danger areas and consciously make a decision to deal with them.

Plan your targets

Everyone works better when working towards a deadline or specific target, and this also applies to a weight-loss programme. If you aim to lose weight for a special occasion, whether it be a wedding or a holiday, you are likely to be infinitely more successful than someone who has no particular goal in mind.

On page 254 you will find a goal chart which should be completed at the outset of your dieting campaign. Set yourself targets for weight loss by a certain day and write alongside the reason why you want to achieve the weight by that date. It's also a good idea to duplicate your goals on a separate little card which you can carry with you at all times as a reminder. Keep it in your purse so that you will continue to notice it during the day and be less likely to be tempted by forbidden foods.

As you achieve each goal you should give yourself a huge reward and ideally involve your partner and the rest of the family in the treat. Only you know what your reward should be, but it should be great enough to inspire you to stick with the diet and exercise programme and to keep your mind on the ultimate goal that you have decided on. By involving the rest of the family, you will find that they will be much more supportive and encouraging of your continuing progress and success.

Measure your progress

Measure yourself on a weekly basis, and you'll be amazed at how quickly the inches disappear on this diet and fitness programme. Record your results on the chart on page 256. Use a tape measure, or try on a tight skirt or pair of trousers and watch and feel how this garment gets looser. Physically seeing those inches disappearing, either by the reducing of the tape measure or the gaps appearing in the waistband of the trousers or skirt, will be a real source on encouragement, so do take the time to do it. Keep that measuring garment specifically for that job and do not wear it at any other time otherwise it will stretch and become artificially loose.

Take a photograph

While no-one feels very confident when they start out on a diet, it is really important to have photographic evidence of how you looked in your 'before' state. Ask a close friend or a partner to be photographer and be quite open about the purpose of the picture. Take a front and side view and wear something that shows you as you really are rather than a garment that flatters you.

You don't necessarily have to look at the photograph until you have lost a significant amount of weight. Ideally, get someone to take a photograph of you as you lose each stone so that you can compare the difference and see your progress. Don't be too disheartened if the first two sets of photographs do not show a vast difference. As time progresses, you will be delighted when you see the difference between how you are now and how you are, say, in three months' time.

Keep a graph

Draw up a graph that you can fill in as you lose each stone (see sample graph on page 258). Use a separate sheet for each stone so that the downward trend looks more dramatic – and more encouraging.

One cheat does not mean failure

Temptation is all around us – from other people, television and advertising, as well as on every shelf of every supermarket or food store that we visit. Every time we buy petrol we are faced with an array of sweets and chocolates as we go to pay for it.

Other family members may start nibbling in between meals and you feel tempted to join in. At your workplace you find that it is somebody's birthday and they treat everyone to a cream cake. Obviously, you would feel embarrassed if you didn't join in. These situations are normal and they don't help us to stick to a diet. We therefore have to come to a compromise.

There are occasions when it is wholly appropriate for you to break the diet and eat something that is not allowed. A cream cake on someone's birthday is a classic example. On such occasions I am all for you joining in and being part of the crowd. Enjoy the cake, don't feel guilty about it and just get back on the diet for the rest of the day and thereafter. Hopefully, there won't be too many birthdays in the next few weeks! I wouldn't class eating a cream cake on a colleague's birthday as a cheat, I would call it a treat. There will be other less justifiable occasions when you just can't resist eating something you shouldn't. You won't necessarily even be feeling hungry when you eat it but, at that particular moment, temptation gets the better of you and the attraction of that chocolate bar or biscuit is just too great. Just because you gave in on that occasion doesn't mean you will do it all the time, so don't categorise yourself as a failure, an uncontrollable cheat, or even a gannet!

Remember, one biscuit will hardly make a difference to your weight loss over a week. The problem comes when you convince yourself that you are likely to cheat again so you might as well eat the whole packet and get them out of the way! That's when the damage is really done.

Create a contingency plan

Whenever you know that you have overindulged, take active steps to counteract the damage that you might have done. The best way to do this is to step up your activity level. This not only increases your energy output and burns calories, but it also has the psychological effect of making you feel that you have done something to counteract your indulgence. Such positive action will, in turn, prevent you from cheating further which could lead to a wholesale binge – something to be avoided at all costs, as bingeing can seriously damage your progress on the diet.

Look at your appearance

As you slim down and tone up, think about changing your image and perhaps wearing styles of clothes that you may not have considered previously because of your shape. Look carefully at your hair and make-up, too. There is no time like the present when it comes to combining the whole package of getting trimmer, increasing our fitness levels and revamping our appearance.

Take the time and trouble to wash and style your hair regularly, consider using make-up if you don't already and carefully coordinate your clothes every day, not just for special occasions. Soon your confidence will build and the compliments will flow as your family and friends notice how much better you look and feel. Success breeds success, and if you look as though you are succeeding, believe me, it will really help you to reach your goal. The other great plus is that once you have got into the habit of making that extra effort with your appearance, this will motivate you to keep slim and looking your best at all times. You will like your new image and that will be the best insurance policy you have for maintaining your new slim figure.

Slim with others

If there is a Rosemary Conley Diet & Fitness Club near you, do go along and join. You will find people just like you, eager to help and support each other in reaching the common goal of a slim and fit body. Having that weekly goal of a weigh-in at a certain time on a certain day is an excellent motivation to keep you on the straight and narrow for a period of seven days at a time. All the instructors are carefully selected by myself and they offer a very special service. They are extensively trained and are qualified exercise teachers who are able to adapt exercises to suit everybody, no matter what their age or activity level. The successes enjoyed at those classes is phenomenal, and I can only encourage you to join the many thousands who have already benefited.

Plan to win

Adopting a positive attitude is essential if you are going to be successful on your diet and fitness campaign. Consciously make an effort to rid your mind of any negative thoughts of possible failure and develop the habit of assertiveness about your intentions of success. If you can actually see yourself succeeding and honestly believe that you can succeed, then you will.

When you have doubts in your mind, you are basically feeding your mind with negative thoughts which could cause you to fail. Fill your mind with positive and successful thoughts and you will be feeding your mind with good and positive images of how you are going to look and feel once you have lost your excess weight.

Be persistent

Failure cannot live with persistence, so, providing you keep trying, you cannot fail. Nobody can dictate how fast you will lose your unwanted weight or how quickly you will get fit or reshape your body, but what I do know for sure is that those who persevere will get there and those who don't bother definitely won't. If you think you'll fail, you will fail, but if you believe you will succeed, you'll win.

5

The New Body Diet

Most people want a trim and healthy body, but we are what we eat and often we eat too much of the wrong things. We need to eat enough of the right things and eat a variety of foods to ensure that we are getting all the necessary nutrients for a healthy, balanced diet.

Getting the balance right in your diet

There are five major food groups: carbohydrate, protein, fat, vitamins and minerals. All these foods form part of a healthy diet, but we need them in varying quantities.

Carbohydrate – potatoes, pasta, rice, cereals, bread – should form the bulk of our diet. These are energy-giving foods that are not readily stored as fat *unless eaten in excess*. Please note those last four words! If we eat too much of anything, we will store it as fat, so if we want to lose weight, obviously we need to moderate our intake. Having said that, the majority of

calories within any of my diets will be from carbohydrate foods. This makes my diets suitable for
diabetics who need regular supplies of carbohydrate
to maintain their insulin levels.

Protein foods are very important, too, as we need
protein for growth and repair. Protein is found in
foods such as meat, fish, eggs, cheese, poultry, milk
and dairy products. However, we only need moderate amounts, though we do need milk for its calcium
content.

Fat is another tangible nutrient, but it is required in
such tiny quantities that, providing we eat a variety of
foods where fat is found quite naturally, we will be
eating sufficient fat without having to add any extra.
Examples of foods that contain beneficial fats are oily
fish such as salmon, tuna and mackerel. While some
of these do contain more than my ruling of four per
cent fat, they do contain valuable nutrients which
play a valuable role in a healthy diet. Where we can
make some economies on fat, though, is in the area of
butter, margarine, cream, oil – the fats that we tend to
add to food. If you don't add any fat, you will automatically be eating a low-fat diet, and eating low fat
will give you a leaner body.

The remaining two food groups – vitamins and
minerals – are intangible. In other words, vitamins
and minerals are found within other foods. For
instance, a potato, which is a carbohydrate, also
contains vitamin C; red meat, which is protein, also
contains iron, and so on. So, vitamins and minerals
complement the other nutrients and are absolutely
vital for good health. By eating a variety of different

foods we can be sure of getting sufficient vitamins and minerals. However, if there is one particular food group that you cannot tolerate, because you simply don't like the taste or you suffer an allergic reaction, you should seek advice on taking that particular nutrient in supplement form.

Within my eating plans I always include foods rich in nutrients to ensure that my dieters eat healthily. My New Body Plan incorporates a free choice diet, because the most successful slimmers will be those people who eat foods that they enjoy. This way, they do not tire of the diet and start eating the wrong foods. It is essential that each individual finds the right formula, which is why most of my diets are designed in such a way that you can choose what you like to eat.

The beauty of this New Body Diet is its total versatility. In addition to three main meals a day you are allowed three snacks. These snacks can be eaten on their own at any time of the day or added on to a breakfast, lunch or dinner menu. Alternatively, if you wish, you could combine your three daily snacks to form an additional meal. Some people may prefer six meals, some three. I am a great advocate of the three-meals-a-day regime, as I feel it establishes a habit that fits in with most lifestyles, but I do understand that some people find it difficult to 'last' between meals.

Do make sure you stick to the quantities I have specified at mealtimes. If you start eating larger quantities for your main meals and still have the snacks, I'm afraid you will not enjoy such a great weight loss.

How to read nutrition labels

We are now fortunate that the nutrient content of most food products is displayed on the packaging. This is of tremendous help to anyone who is watching their weight and their health.

As far as weight control is concerned, there are only two details you need to read carefully on the label: the 'energy' value and the 'fat' content. The energy value will be shown in kilojoules or kilocalories – kJ or kcal for short. The 'kcal' figure will tell you the number of calories per 100 grams.

The fat content may be split as follows:

FAT	4 g
of which saturates	2.5 g
unsaturates	1.5 g

This means that within 100 grams of this product there are four grams of fat. The fat is of two types, saturated (mainly animal origin) and unsaturated (plant or fish origin). On a low-fat, weight-reducing diet, however, it's irrelevant where the fat comes from, so you can ignore the finer detail. All you need to know is the total fat content. As a general rule, when selecting foods in the supermarket, choose only those foods that contain four grams or less per 100 grams of the product. That's equivalent to four per cent fat. Read labels carefully, particularly when foods are labelled 'lite' or 'reduced fat'. Many so called low-fat spreads and dressings still contain large amounts of fat, so make sure you always check the nutrition panel carefully.

While the four per cent rule is a good yardstick, there are exceptions. If you remove the skin and all visible fat, then lean beef, lamb, pork, venison, poultry and fish are totally acceptable. The other exceptions are products such as mustard, curry powder, and so on, where you will only be eating minimal amounts. Use your discretion.

How to make the New Body Plan work for you

1 Decide on your menu plan for the day. It's a good idea to keep a food diary and record everything you eat and drink. So, as you eat each meal or snack, write down exactly what you do eat so that you can accurately gauge what you ate and when. Once you are familiar with your favourite meals and recipes and what time of day you actually eat rather than when you think you eat, you can plan future meals more easily.

2 Be sure to eat at least three meals a day and don't skip breakfast. Breakfast should be eaten before 10am.

3 Fill up at mealtimes to satisfy your appetite by eating lots of low-calorie salads or boiled, steamed or raw vegetables (excluding potatoes).

4 Have a long, low-calorie drink before each mealtime and during each meal to help fill you up.

5 Drink as much water as you can. This is good for your health, helps you to feel full more quickly and prevents dehydration.

6 If you receive an unexpected invitation to a meal,

try to choose what you eat carefully and cut out the snacks the next day.

7 If on one day you have an absolute cheat – say a bar of chocolate – don't abandon the diet and think that you have undone all the good that you have done so far. You won't have, but please do stop after the one indiscretion and don't go on to eat another six bars. Remember, additional exercise will help to burn off those extra calories, and the last thing I want you to do is to get hung up on the fact that you have had a bit of a cheat. It is the overall picture that matters. Work out for an extra 20 minutes on the day you overdo the calories.

8 Remember, to maximise your fat loss you need to combine low-fat fat eating with regular exercise, so follow my New Body Workout in Chapter 7, which includes both toning and aerobic exercises. In addition to practising these exercises at least three times a week, try to be more physically active in your everyday life. Park your car at the furthest space from your office or the supermarket. Step up the pace as you walk, and don't hesitate to run upstairs at the slightest excuse.

9 Please do get someone to take a photograph of you before and after your weight-loss campaign. You don't have to show the 'before' photograph to anybody, and it can be hidden away at the bottom of a drawer. When you've lost your excess weight and can see the amazing progress that you have made before and after your weight loss campaign, you'll be so glad you took that photograph.

10 Take the time to weigh yourself each week at the same time of day, wearing the same clothes and using the same scales. Measure yourself, too, using a tape measure or a measuring garment such as a tight pair of trousers or a skirt. Ideally get your partner to help you with your weighing and measuring session. When they see you benefiting, they will feel part of the success. Everyone likes to feel needed, and your partner's encouragement is particularly important towards the end of your weight-loss campaign.

Diet instructions

Each day you are allowed a breakfast, lunch and dinner, which should be taken from the selections listed. Then you have a choice. In addition to these three meals, you may select a mid-morning, a mid-afternoon and a mid-evening snack from the appropriate lists (see pages 75–78). These snacks may be eaten either between meals or at mealtimes if you prefer. Or you could combine your three snacks to form an additional meal. Adapt the diet to suit you, but do eat your allocation of food to ensure the maintenance of your metabolic rate and the ability of your body to use its fat stores to supplement the calories supplied. If you eat less than the amounts specified, you may find that your metabolism slows down.

For this diet to be effective for you you have to make it fit your lifestyle pattern. The only basic rule that must be adhered to is that you must eat at least three meals a day and do not skip meals.

The calorie content of this diet is around 1400 a day. Check your weight, age and activity level against the metabolic chart (see pages 10–12) to find out your personal calorie allowance. Add additional calories, if appropriate, by eating extra fruit or by increasing your serving sizes of pasta, rice or potatoes. If you need to increase the number of calories, carbohydrate is the best choice.

All foods included in this diet contain a maximum of four per cent fat unless the quantity of food is so small that the total fat content is insignificant. Vegetarians will find that some additional oil has been included to compensate for the fact that they will not be consuming fat from meat.

It is essential that you do not eat any foods from the list overleaf. Otherwise, your rate of progress in terms of both weight and inches will inevitably slow down and you may in fact gain weight. Remember that eating too much of anything can cause you to gain weight, so if your progress appears too slow, do check the quantities of food you are eating.

Don't eat these foods if you want to lose weight

If you want to lose weight and inches, then do not eat the following foods, unless they are specifically included in the diet menus or recipes. Exceptions are made only for vegetarians who may include a little low-fat cheese, additional eggs and a few drops of oil in their cooking.

Avocado pears and olives

Butter, margarine, low-fat spreads, mayonnaise

Cakes, biscuits, pastries, quiches, egg custard, crackers, marzipan, sponge puddings etc

Cheese: all varieties including low-fat brands, except cottage cheese

Chocolate, toffees, fudge, caramel, butterscotch

Cream, cream cheese, soured cream, cream from full-fat milk

Crisps and snacks

Desserts made from cream, such as crème brûlée, crème caramel, home-made ice-cream

Dressings, sauces containing more than four per cent fat

Fats and oils, e.g. cooking oil, lard, dripping, suet, fat from meat

Fatty meats, e.g. goose

Fried foods of any kind (except dry-fried)

Full-fat yogurts, Greek yogurt (check the label for fat content)

Horlicks, drinking chocolate, cocoa and cocoa products

Lemon curd, peanut butter, chocolate spread

Meat products such as Scotch eggs, pork pies, faggots, black pudding, haggis, pâté, salami, sausages, skin from all meats and poultry

Diet notes

Bread should be wholemeal whenever possible. For guidance, one slice of regular bread from a large thin-sliced loaf weighs 25g (1oz). A slice from a large medium-sliced loaf weighs 40g (1½oz). Unless otherwise specified in the menus, one slice equals 25g (1oz). Light bread means low-calorie brands such as Nimble or St Michael's Lite bread.

Cottage cheese should be the low-fat variety. Flavoured varieties are acceptable, but check the nutritional panel for fat content and avoid ones with added cream.

Diet yogurt means low-fat, low-calorie brands. 1 x 150g (5oz) pot should contain no more than 70 calories.

Gravy may be taken with the dinner menus, provided it is made with gravy powder or low-fat granules. Do not add meat juices from the roasting tin unless you first discard the fat.

1 piece fresh fruit means one average apple or one orange etc. or approximately 115g (4oz) of any fruit such as grapes, pineapple, strawberries etc. Do not eat fruit between meals except as part of a prescribed snack.

Pasta and rice are restricted to 50g (2oz) dry weight per portion unless otherwise specified. 50g (2oz) dry weight rice weighs 150g (5oz) when cooked, and 50g (2oz) dry weight pasta weighs 175g (6oz). Choose wholemeal varieties where possible. Always boil without adding oil or fat. Unlimited quantities of canned or fresh beansprouts may be added to bulk up small quantities of rice.

Unlimited vegetables includes all vegetables (with the exception of potatoes), providing they are cooked and served without fat. In this diet, potatoes are excluded from this section because of the additional snacks allowed.

Sauces and dressings

The following may be consumed freely:

Brown sauce	Mustard
Chilli sauce	Oil-free vinaigrette
Fat-free salad dressings	Soy sauce
Horseradish sauce	Tomato ketchup
Lemon juice	Vinegar (any type)
Marmite	Worcester sauce
Mint sauce	

For other sauces and dressings check the nutrition panel on the label before you buy and only select those with four per cent or less fat, except for items of which you will consume only minimal amounts.

Daily allowance

- 450ml (¾ pint) skimmed or semi-skimmed milk
- One unit alcoholic drink for women, two for men
- Tea and coffee may be drunk freely, using milk from allowance. Diet drinks and water are also unlimited
- Unlimited salad with fat-free dressing may be served with lunch and dinner.

Note

All branded products included in this diet were available at the time of going to press, but manufacturers' ranges are subject to change.

The New Body Diet

BREAKFASTS
Cereal breakfasts
Fruit breakfasts
Quick and easy breakfasts
Cooked breakfasts

LUNCHES
Quick and easy lunches
Home-made sandwiches
Pre-packed sandwiches
Salads
Soups
Gourmet lunches

DINNERS
Quick and easy main courses
Cooking sauce main courses
Ready-made main courses: meat, poultry and fish
Ready-made main courses: vegetarian
Gourmet main courses: meat and poultry
Gourmet main courses: fish
Gourmet main courses: vegetarian
Side dishes

DESSERTS
Quick and easy desserts
Gourmet desserts

SNACKS
Mid-morning and supper snacks
Mid-afternoon snacks

Breakfasts

Select any one.

Cereal breakfasts

Serve with milk from allowance.

- 40g (1½oz) any cereal with 2 teaspoons sugar.
- 25g (1oz) any cereal with 1 teaspoon sugar, plus 1 piece fresh fruit.
- 25g (1oz) muesli, plus 115g (4oz) sliced strawberries or ½ banana, sliced.
- 25g (1oz) muesli mixed with 150g (5oz) low-fat yogurt.
- 40g (1½oz) sultana bran with 1 teaspoon sugar.
- 50g (2oz) Kellogg's All-Bran with 2 teaspoons sugar.
- 50g (2oz) Kellogg's Frosties.
- 50g (2oz) Kellogg's Rice Krispies with 1 teaspoon sugar.
- 2 Weetabix with 2 teaspoons sugar.
- 50g (2oz) St Michael Multi Flake Cereal, plus 1 piece fresh fruit.

Fruit breakfasts

- 4 pieces fresh fruit, e.g. 1 banana, 1 apple, 1 pear, 1 orange.
- 115g (4oz) any stewed fruit cooked without sugar or 115g (4oz) canned fruit in natural juice, topped with 1 x 150g (5oz) diet yogurt.
- 2 pieces fresh fruit, plus 1 x 150g (5oz) diet yogurt.
- 2 slices fresh pineapple, plus 1 x 150g (5oz) pineapple-flavoured diet yogurt.

- 1 fruit platter made with sliced melon, kiwi fruit, oranges, apples and banana (maximum total weight 450g/1lb).
- 225g (8oz) canned grapefruit segments in natural juice.
- ½ Galia melon, topped with 115g (4oz) strawberries.
- 350g (12oz) fresh fruit salad topped with 150g (5oz) diet yogurt.
- 1 x 200g pack St Michael Autumn Fruit Salad, topped with 1 tablespoon low-fat yogurt.
- 1 x 175g pack St Michael Fruit Cocktail, topped with 1 x 150g pot St Michael Very Low Fat Lite Yoghurt.
- 1 St Michael Very Low Fat Lite Yoghurt and Fruit twinpot, plus 1 apple.

Quick and easy breakfasts

- 1 whole fresh grapefruit, 1 boiled egg, and 1 Ryvita spread with Marmite.
- 1 slice (40g/1½oz) wholemeal toast spread with 2 teaspoons marmalade, plus 1 piece fresh fruit.
- 2 slices light wholemeal bread (e.g. St Michael Lite Bread) or similar spread with 2 teaspoons marmalade or preserve, plus 1 apple or orange.
- 1 slice (40g/1½oz) wholemeal toast spread with Marmite and topped with 50g (2oz) low-fat cottage cheese.
- 1 slice (40g/1½oz) wholemeal toast spread thinly with mustard and topped with 50g (2oz) wafer thin ham or turkey or beef.

- 2 slices light wholemeal bread spread with horseradish sauce and filled with 25g (1oz) pastrami.
- 2 St Michael Pikelets, topped with 2 teaspoons raspberry conserve and 2 tablespoons low-fat fromage frais.

Cooked breakfasts

- 25g (1oz) [dry weight] porridge cooked in water and served with 1 teaspoon honey plus milk from allowance.
- ½ fresh grapefruit, plus 1 slice light wholemeal toast topped with 2 grilled turkey rashers (e.g. Mattesons) plus 2 sliced tomatoes.
- 1 slice light wholemeal bread, toasted and topped with 1 x 200g (7oz) can tomatoes which have been well boiled and reduced to a creamy consistency and 1 grilled turkey rasher.
- 1 slice light bread, toasted and topped with 1 x 200g (7oz) can baked beans.
- 2 slices light wholemeal bread, toasted and spread with HP or Branston Fruity Sauce and made into a sandwich with 1 grilled turkey rasher and sliced tomato.
- 2 grilled turkey rashers and unlimited grilled tomatoes and mushrooms cooked without fat, plus 1 slice light wholemeal bread, toasted.

Lunches

Select any one.

Quick and easy lunches

- 1 cup instant soup, plus 1 x 25g (1oz) small bread roll (e.g. St Michael Mini Roll), plus 1 x 100g pot St Michael Lite Fromage Frais and 1 banana.
- 2 x 25g (2 x 1oz) small bread rolls spread with Branston or similar pickle and filled with 50g (2oz) wafer thin ham, turkey, chicken or pork, plus 1 piece fresh fruit or 1 cup instant soup.
- Omelette made with 1 egg and milk from allowance. Add a selection of cooked vegetables such as peas, sweetcorn, chopped peppers, and dry-fried chopped onion. Season well with black pepper and serve with unlimited cherry tomatoes.
- 5 pieces any fresh fruit.
- 2 bananas, plus 200g (7oz) low-fat fromage frais.
- 2 slices light bread, toasted and topped with 1 x 200g (7oz) can baked beans.
- 1 slice light bread, toasted and topped with 1 x 200g (7oz) can baked beans plus 1 grilled turkey rasher and sliced tomatoes.
- 1 x 175g (6oz) jacket potato, topped with 50g (2oz) tuna or low-fat cottage cheese and served with unlimited salad.
- 1 x 175g (6oz) jacket potato, topped with 115g (4oz) baked beans and served with unlimited salad.
- 1 x 175g (6oz) jacket potato, topped with 50g (2oz) low-fat cottage cheese mixed with 1 tablespoon

low-fat salad dressing and 1 tablespoon sweetcorn
and chopped peppers, plus unlimited salad.

- 1 x 420g pack St Michael crudités with soured
cream and chive dip.
- 3 x 100g pots St Michael Lite Natural Fromage
Frais, mixed with 115g (4oz) St Michael Summer
Fruits Compote.
- 1 x 200g pack St Michael Autumn Fruit Salad,
topped with 1 x 100g pot St Michael Lite Natural
Fromage Frais.
- 1 x 175g pack St Michael Fruit Cocktail Fresh
Fruit Salad Prepared in a Light Syrup, topped with
1 x 100g pot St Michael Lite Natural Fromage
Frais.
- 1 St Michael Low Fat Ready to Eat Skinless,
Boneless Chicken Breast Fillet, served with 1 x
190g pack St Michael Cherry Tomato Salad, plus 1
St Michael Lite Mousse, any flavour.
- ½ x 230g pack St Michael Lime and Coriander
Chicken Mini Fillets, served with unlimited salad.
- 1 x 250g pack St Michael Vegetable Stir Fry.
- ½ x 320g pack St Michael Italian Style Tuna
Balsamic, served with 115g (4oz) potatoes or 65g
(2½oz) [dry weight] boiled rice, plus unlimited
vegetables.
- ½ x 260g pack St Michael Italian Style Chicken
Piccante, served with 115g (4oz) potatoes and
unlimited vegetables.
- 1 x 400g can Weight Watchers from Heinz Italiana
Tuna Twists.
- 1 x 400g can Weight Watchers from Heinz Italiana
Tortellini.

- 1 x 390g can Weight Watchers from Heinz Italiana Vegetable Ravioli in Chunky Tomato Sauce.

Home-made sandwiches

- 2 slices (2 x 40g/1½oz) wholemeal bread spread with low-fat dressing, sauce or pickle and made into a sandwich with 50g (2oz) low-fat cottage cheese or tuna (in brine) or 50g (2oz) wafer thin ham, chicken or turkey, plus unlimited salad.
- 2 slices light bread spread with Marmite and filled with 50g (2oz) low-fat cottage cheese and unlimited salad.
- 2 slices light bread spread with low-fat salad dressing and filled with 25g (1oz) wafer thin chicken or ham plus 25g (1oz) low-fat cottage cheese and unlimited salad.
- 2 slices light bread toasted and spread with Branston or HP Fruity Sauce and made into a sandwich with 2 grilled turkey rashers and sliced tomatoes.
- 1 pitta bread slit open and spread with low-fat Marie Rose sauce and filled with shredded lettuce and 50g (2oz) cooked and shelled prawns.
- 1 pitta bread slit open and spread with Weight Watchers from Heinz Blue Cheese Flavoured Low Fat Dressing and filled with shredded lettuce and 50g (2oz) low-fat cottage cheese mixed with chopped green and red peppers.
- 1 pitta bread slit open and spread with low-fat dressing and filled with shredded lettuce and 25g

(1oz) shredded wafer thin turkey, beef, chicken or
ham, topped with chopped tomatoes.
- 1 pitta bread slit open and spread with low-fat
  dressing and filled with shredded lettuce and
  50g (2oz) wafer thin chicken, turkey or ham.

Prepacked sandwiches

1 pack of any of the following, plus 1 piece fresh fruit.
- Boots Shapers Turkey and Chinese Leaf.
- Boots Shapers Smoked Ham, Soft Cheese and
  Pineapple.
- Boots Shapers Salmon and Cucumber.
- Boots Shapers Tuna and Cucumber.
- Boots Shapers Prawn, Apple and Celery.
- Boots Shapers Ham Salad.
- Sainsbury's Oriental Style Prawn and Vegetable
  Salad.
- Sainsbury's Chicken Salad.
- Sainsbury's Ham Salad.
- Sainsbury's Turkey Salad.
- Sainsbury's Tuna Salad.
- St Michael Chicken and Lemon Mayonnaise
  with Lettuce and Watercress on Wholemeal
  Bread.
- St Michael Lean Danish Ham and Salad with
  Mustard Dressing on Oatmeal Bread.
- St Michael Wafer Thin Smoked Turkey and
  Coleslaw.
- St Michael Egg and Salad.
- St Michael Tuna and Salad.
- Tesco Red Salmon and Cucumber.

Salads

- Large mixed salad, served with 115g (4oz) low-fat cottage cheese or 50g (2oz) wafer thin ham, chicken, turkey, beef or pastrami, reduced-oil salad dressing, plus 1 x 25g (1oz) small bread roll (e.g. St Michael Mini Roll).
- 25g (1oz) [dry weight] brown rice, cooked and mixed with 50g (2oz) canned chick peas, 25g (1oz) canned red kidney beans, 2 tablespoons cooked peas, 2 tablespoons sweetcorn and unlimited chopped peppers, chopped tomatoes, diced cucumber and spring onions. Serve on a bed of lettuce with fat-free dressing of your choice.
- Prawn Salad (page 83).
- Sardine, Beetroot and Red Apple Salad (page 85).
- Kipper Salad (page 85).
- Prawn and Mango Salad (page 84).
- Crispy Vegetable Salad (page 86).
- Fruit and Chicken Salad (page 87).
- 1 pack St Michael New Potato and Egg Salad, plus additional salad.
- 1 x 190g pack St Michael Couscous and Chargrilled Vegetable Salad, plus 1 slice bread and 1 x 150g (5oz) diet yogurt.
- ½ x 450g pack St Michael Reduced Fat Layered Salad with Prawns.
- 1 pack St Michael Prepared Salad Vegetables sprinkled with low-fat salad dressing, plus 50g (2oz) wafer thin ham, chicken, turkey or beef and 1 x 25g (1oz) small bread roll spread with low-fat salad dressing.

- 1 pack St Michael Reduced Fat Layered Salad with Chicken, plus unlimited green salad and 1 piece fresh fruit.
- 115g (4oz) wafer thin meat of your choice plus one of the following:
  - 1 x 200g pack St Michael New Potato and Tomato Salad
  - 1 x 180g pack St Michael Green Salad
  - 1 x 230g pack St Michael Crunchy Salad with Apple
  - 1 x 190g pack St Michael Cherry Tomato Salad.

Soups

- 300ml (½ pint) Bean Soup (page 80).
- 300ml (½ pint) Red Lentil Soup (page 81).
- 300ml (½ pint) Vegetable Soup (page 82).
- 1 x 425g can Baxters Healthy Choice Lentil and Vegetable Soup, plus 1 slice light bread.
- ½ x 425g can Baxters Carrot and Butterbean Soup, plus 1 banana or 1 slice bread.
- ½ x 425g can Baxters Lobster Bisque, plus 1 slice (40g/1½oz) wholemeal toast.
- 1 x 295g can Campbell's Condensed Half Fat Mushroom Soup reconstituted with water, plus 1 slice bread.
- 1 x 392g can Co-op French Onion Soup, plus 1 x 25g (1oz) small bread roll or 1 slice light bread.
- 1 x 425g can St Michael Chunky Meal Soup Chicken and Vegetable, plus 1 piece fresh fruit.
- 1 x 295g can Weight Watchers from Heinz Mediterranean Tomato and Vegetable Soup, plus

2 slices light bread, toasted and spread with
Marmite, and 1 piece fresh fruit.
- 1 x 295g can Weight Watchers from Heinz Carrot
  and Lentil Soup, plus 1 slice (40g/1½oz)
  wholemeal bread and 1 x 150g (5oz) diet yogurt.

Gourmet lunches

- Turkey Rashers with Chilli and Pasta (page 90).
- Crispy Topped Mushrooms (page 88).
- Banana Surprise (page 89).
- Pasta with Spinach Sauce (page 91).
- Savoury Cauliflower Bake (page 89).
- Tuna Burgers (page 92).
- Tuna Fish Pie (page 92).
- Creamy Curried Quorn (page 000).
- Courgette Provençale (page 93).
- Tomato and Cheese Tarts (page 94).
- Red Kidney Bean Curry (page 95).
- Creamy Cauliflower Pasta (page 96).
- Ratatouille au Gratin (page 97).
- Baked Artichokes with Apricots (page 97).
- Toasted Muffin Pizza (page 99).
- Pepper and Wholewheat Pasta (page 99).

Dinners: Main Courses

Select any one.

Quick and easy main courses

- Choice of 175g (6oz) white fish or 115g (4oz) chicken (no skin) or 75g (3oz) red meat, grilled, baked or microwaved. Serve with either 115g (4oz) potatoes or 50g (2oz) [dry weight] rice or pasta, plus unlimited vegetables or salad.
- 1 St Michael Seasoned Tuna Fillet or Fresh Rainbow Trout Fillet, served with 175g (6oz) new potatoes and unlimited vegetables.
- 3 St Michael Extra Lean Pork Sausages (3.7% fat), grilled, and served with 115g (4oz) potatoes and unlimited vegetables.
- 1 x 100g St Michael Low Fat Lightly Smoked Sweetcure Gammon Steak, served with 1 slice pineapple, 175g (6oz) new potatoes and unlimited vegetables.
- 1 x 100g St Michael Unsmoked Sweetcure Honey Glazed Gammon Joint, served with 115g (4oz) new potatoes, unlimited vegetables and fat-free gravy or sauce.
- 1 x 150g St Michael Honey and Mustard Marinaded Chicken Breast Joint, served with 115g (4oz) potatoes and unlimited vegetables.
- 1 x 220g can St Michael Chunky Steak, served with 115g (4oz) potatoes and unlimited vegetables.
- ½ x 300g pack St Michael Low Fat Chargrilled Chicken with Lime and Coriander, served with 175g (6oz) potatoes and unlimited vegetables.

- 1 x 300g pack St Michael Low Fat Chargrilled
  Lemon Chicken, served with 115g (4oz) new
  potatoes and unlimited vegetables.

Cooking sauce main courses

Poultry
Allow 115g (4oz) chicken or turkey per person (men
may have an additional 50g/2oz).

Remove all skin prior to cooking where possible as
the majority of fat in poultry is found in the skin.
Chicken and turkey can be dry-fried in a non-stick pan
without any added moisture. Chop the chicken or
turkey, if necessary. To seal the juices, preheat the pan
and add the poultry in small batches to prevent the pan
cooling during cooking. Turn the poultry regularly for
all-over browning before you add the sauce. If using
chicken or turkey breasts whole, dry-fry in the same
manner to brown, then add the sauce and allow a longer
cooking time to ensure the chicken is thoroughly cooked.

Note 1 x 500g can or jar of sauce serves 4, or allow
125g per person. Serve with 150g (5oz) [cooked
weight] boiled rice or 175g (6oz) [cooked weight]
pasta or 175g (6oz) boiled potatoes, plus unlimited
vegetables.

Add any of the following sauces:
Asda Healthy Choice Korma Balti Curry
Asda Healthy Choice Sweet and Sour Chinese Style
  Stir Fry
Asda Healthy Choice Tikka Masala
Chicken Tonight Barbecue

Chicken Tonight Chinese Bean and Ginger
Chicken Tonight Spanish Chicken
Homepride Creamy Tomato and Tarragon
Patak's Original Dopiaza
Sainsbury's Chicken Saucery Tomato and Pepper
St Michael Black Bean Stir Fry
St Michael Oriental Stir Fry
St Michael Sweet and Sour Stir Fry
Sharwood's Stir Fry Sweet and Sour
Sharwood's Stir Fry Szechuan with Crunchy Vegetables
Uncle Ben's Sweet and Sour Stir Fry
Tesco Sweet and Sour Stir Fry
Waitrose Creole
Waitrose Masala
Weight Watchers from Heinz Low Fat Louisiana
    Cajun
Worldwide Sweet and Sour Stir Fry

Beef, lamb, pork
Allow 115g (4oz) meat per person (men may have an additional 50g/2oz).

Remove any fat before cooking. If using mince, dry-fry in a non stick pan. When the meat has turned brown, drain well through a sieve or colander and wipe any remaining fat from the pan with a kitchen towel. The meat is then ready to be cooked with the sauce and any other ingredients such as onions and mushrooms. For casseroles where diced lean meat is use, the meat will be more tender if added raw, without any pre-cooking.

Note 1 x 500g can or jar of sauce serves 4, or allow 125g per person. Serve with 115g (4oz) boiled potatoes or 115g (4oz) [cooked weight] boiled rice or 150g (5oz) [cooked weight] boiled pasta per person.

Add any of the following sauces:
Homepride Tomato and Onion
Homepride Creamy Garlic and Herb
Ragù Pasta Sauce with Onion and Garlic
Sainsbury's Beef Saucery Red Wine and Herb
St Michael Italian Style Pasta Sauce
Schwartz Thai 7 Spice Stir Fry
Tesco Rogan Josh
Uncle Ben's Light Chilli Con Carne
Weight Watchers from Heinz Chinese Szechuan
Weight Watchers from Heinz Mexican Chilli
Worldwide Madras Curry

Fish
Allow 175g (6oz) any type of fish or seafood per person (men may have an additional 50g/2oz).

Remove any skin and bones and rinse in cold water. Chop into bite-sized chunks and cook according to the instructions on the can or jar, but avoid the use of fat or oil. Some instructions may suggest frying the fish in butter or oil. Instead, dry-fry the fish in a non-stick pan, adding a little water or wine if it becomes too dry. To add more flavour, sprinkle with freshly ground black pepper.

Note 1 x 500g can or jar of sauce serves 4, or allow 125g per person. Serve with 75g (3oz) [cooked weight] boiled rice mixed with unlimited canned beansprouts, or 175g (6oz) boiled potatoes, plus other unlimited boiled vegetables.

Add any of the following sauces:
Sainsbury's Fish Saucery Tomato and Tarragon
Tesco Red Thai Curry Stir Fry

Ready-made main courses: meat, poultry and fish

Asda

- 1 x 350g pack Asda Healthy Choice Lasagne, served with unlimited green salad.
- 1 x 340g pack Asda Healthy Choice Beef Oriental with Rice, served with unlimited vegetables.
- 1 x 340g pack Asda Healthy Choice Chicken in White Wine, served with unlimited vegetables.
- 1 x 300g pack Asda Healthy Choice Chicken Tikka with Rice, served with unlimited salad.
- 1 x 400g pack Asda Chicken Casserole, served with 115g (4oz) mashed potato and unlimited vegetables.
- ½ x 200g pack Asda Chicken, Broccoli and Pasta Bake, served with unlimited vegetables.
- 1 x 400g pack Asda Tagliatelle Carbonara, served with unlimited salad.
- 1 x 300g pack Asda Spaghetti Bolognese, served with unlimited salad.

Birds Eye

- 1 x 368g pack Bird's Eye Healthy Options Glazed Chicken with Duchesse Potatoes, Broccoli Florets and Carrots.

- 1 x 368g pack Birds Eye Healthy Options Steak in Red Wine with Mushrooms, Duchesse Potatoes, Green Beans and Carrots.
- ½ x 400g pack Birds Eye Fish Cuisine Medley Cheese and Broccoli Mornay, served with 115g (4oz) potatoes and unlimited vegetables.

Bistro Menu

- 1 x 300g pack Bistro Menu Fish Linguini, served with unlimited vegetables.
- 1 x 300g pack Bistro Menu Tuna Risotto, served with unlimited vegetables.

Findus Lean Cuisine

- 1 x 230g pack Findus Lean Cuisine Spanish Paella, served with unlimited vegetables.
- 1 x 272g pack Findus Lean Cuisine Glazed Chicken with Rice, served with unlimited vegetables.
- 1 x 230g pack Findus Lean Cuisine Smoked Ham and Mushroom Tagliatelle, served with unlimited vegetables.

Ken Hom

- ½ x 375g pack Ken Hom Cuisine Sweet and Sour Chicken with Sesame Rice, served with unlimited vegetables or salad.

Safeway

- 1 x 300g pack Safeway Chicken Curry, served with unlimited vegetables.
- 1 x 300g pack Safeway Beef Curry with Rice, served with unlimited vegetables.

- $\frac{1}{2}$ x 460g pack Safeway Corned Beef Hash, served with unlimited vegetables.
- 1 x 300g pack Sainsbury's Minced Beef Casserole, served with unlimited vegetables.
- 1 x 300g pack Sainsbury's Chilli Con Carne with Rice, served with unlimited vegetables.
- $\frac{1}{2}$ x 520g pack Sainsbury's Lancashire Hotpot, served with unlimited vegetables.
- 1 x 300g pack Sainsbury's Chicken Chow Mein, served with unlimited vegetables.
- $\frac{1}{2}$ x 300g pack Sainsbury's Sweet and Sour Chicken, served with 150g (5oz) [cooked weight] rice.

St Michael
- $\frac{1}{2}$ x 480g pack St Michael Chilli Con Carne with Rice, served with unlimited salad.
- 1 x 283g pack St Michael Shanghai Shredded Meats, served with 65g (2½oz) [cooked weight] rice.
- 1 x 200g pack St Michael Sweet and Sour Pork, served with unlimited vegetables.
- $\frac{1}{2}$ x 390g pack St Michael Reduced Fat Lite Pork Fillet in a Light Mustard Sauce, served with 115g (4oz) potatoes and unlimited vegetables.
- 1 x 283g pack St Michael Low Fat Lasagne, served with unlimited vegetables or salad.
- 1 x 250g pack St Michael Reduced Fat Lite Chicken Broccoli and Tomato, served with unlimited vegetables.
- $\frac{1}{2}$ x 483g pack St Michael Chicken Sag with Basmati Rice, served with unlimited salad.

- ½ x 320g pack St Michael Chicken with Carrot and Orange, served with 115g (4oz) potatoes and unlimited vegetables.
- 1 x 340g pack St Michael Chicken Couscous, served with unlimited vegetables.
- ½ x 300g pack St Michael Tuna Steak with Sweet Pepper, Coriander and Lime Topping, served with 115g (4oz) potatoes and unlimited vegetables.
- 1 x 340g pack St Michael Prawn Balti, served with 65g (2½oz) [cooked weight] rice.
- 1 x 300g pack St Michael Haddock Meuniere with Vegetables Meal For One, served with unlimited vegetables.
- 1 x 380g pack St Michael Lite Low Fat Smoked Haddock Meal, served with unlimited vegetables.
- ½ x 510g pack St Michael Haddock and Parsley Bake, served with unlimited vegetables.

Tesco
- 1 x 340g pack Tesco Seafood Provençale, served with 115g (4oz) potatoes and unlimited vegetables.
- ½ x 400g Tesco Gobi Aloo Sag, served with 50g (2oz) [cooked weight] rice.
- 1 x 370g pack Tesco Chicken in Black Bean Sauce with Egg Rice, served with unlimited green salad.
- 1 x 370g pack Tesco Beef with Ginger and Spring Onions with Egg Rice, served with unlimited vegetables.

Tiffany's
- 1 x 325g pack Tiffany's Value Master Sweet and Sour Chicken with Rice, served with unlimited vegetables.

Weight Watchers from Heinz
- 1 x 300g pack Weight Watchers from Heinz Chicken Supreme with Rice.
- 1 x 290g pack Weight Watchers from Heinz Chicken in Peppercorn Sauce, served with unlimited vegetables.
- 1 x 305g pack Weight Watchers from Heinz Chicken and Broccoli Pasta Bake, served with unlimited vegetables.
- 1 x 300g pack Weight Watchers from Heinz Chicken Curry with Rice, served with unlimited vegetables.
- 1 x 295g pack Weight Watchers from Heinz Beef Lasagne, served with unlimited salad.
- 1 x 320g pack Weight Watchers from Heinz Lincolnshire Sausage and Bean Hotpot, served with unlimited vegetables.
- 1 x 300g pack Weight Watchers from Heinz Mexican Chilli with Potato Wedges, served with unlimited vegetables.
- 1 x 400g can Weight Watchers from Heinz Italiana Pasta Tubes, served with unlimited vegetables.
- 1 x 400g can Weight Watchers from Heinz Italiana Bolognese shells, served with unlimited vegetables.
- 1 x 300g pack Weight Watchers from Heinz Tagliatelle Carbonara, served with unlimited vegetables.

- 1 x 295g pack Weight Watchers from Heinz Ocean Pie, served with unlimited vegetables.
- 1 x 320g pack Weight Watchers from Heinz Salmon and Prawn Tagliatelle, served with unlimited vegetables.
- 1 x 290g pack Weight Watchers from Heinz Salmon Mornay with Broccoli, served with unlimited vegetables.
- 1 x 320g pack Weight Watchers from Heinz Pasta Niçoise with Tuna, served with unlimited vegetables.
- 1 x 320g pack Weight Watchers from Heinz Spinach and Ricotta Pasta with Smoked Ham, served with unlimited vegetables.
- 1 x 320g pack Weight Watchers from Heinz Chicken Rogan Josh with Vegetable Rice, served with unlimited vegetables.
- 1 x 320g pack Weight Watchers from Heinz Chicken Dopiaza with Vegetable Rice, served with unlimited vegetables.
- 1 x 290g pack Weight Watchers from Heinz Chicken Korma with Rice, served with unlimited vegetables.

Readymade main course dishes: vegetarian

- 1 x 300g pack Asda Vegetable and Lentil Hash, served with unlimited vegetables.
- 1 x 230g pack Findus Lean Cuisine Vegetable Tikka Masala, served with unlimited salad.
- 1 x 250g pack Sainsbury's Vegetarian Pasta Bake, served with unlimited vegetables.

- 1 x 300g pack Sainsbury's Vegetarian Cottage Pie, served with unlimited vegetables.
- 1 x 250g pack Sainsbury's Vegetarian Rigatoni Arrabiata, served with unlimited vegetables.
- 1 x 250g pack Sainsbury's Vegetable Chilli, served with unlimited vegetables.
- 1 x 283g pack St Michael Fresh Vegetable Ratatouille, served with 175g (6oz) [cooked weight] brown rice.
- ½ x 450g pack St Michael Fresh Vegetable Bake, served with unlimited vegetables.
- ½ St Michael Lite Fresh Vegetable Pizza, served with unlimited salad.
- 1 x 283g pack St Michael Fresh Filled Green Pepper, served with unlimited vegetables.
- 1 x 340g pack St Michael Low Fat Fresh Tikka Masala with Indian Rice, served with unlimited vegetables.
- 1 x 454g pack St Michael Low Fat Vegetable Indian Meal.
- 1 x 283g pack St Michael Low Fat Fresh Vegetable and Bean Chilli, served with 175g (6oz) [cooked weight] rice.
- 1 x 320g pack Weight Watchers from Heinz Vegetable Lasagne, served with unlimited vegetables.
- 1 x 320g pack Weight Watchers from Heinz Vegetable and Pasta Medley, served with unlimited vegetables.
- 1 x 335g pack Weight Watchers from Heinz Vegetable Hotpot, served with unlimited vegetables.

- 1 x 320g pack Weight Watchers from Heinz
  Vegetable Balti with Naan Bread, served with
  unlimited vegetables.

Gourmet main courses: meat and poultry

- Lamb Burgers (page 100).
- Lamb and Pineapple Curry (page 101).
- Savoury Lamb Mince (page 102).
- Faggots with Gravy (page 103).
- Autumn Country Bake (page 104).
- Beef and Orange Curry (page 105).
- Mince and Ginger Stir-fry (page 106).
- Bacon and Runner Bean Stir-fry (page 107).
- Italian-style Gammon Steaks (page 107).
- Leek and Ham Cannelloni (page 108).
- Savoury Rice with Ham (page 109).
- Chinese Pork with Ginger (page 110).
- Gingered Pork with Apricots (page 110).
- Pork and Apple Parcels (page 111).
- Pork Crumble (page 112).
- Pork Stroganoff (page 113).
- Zingy Limed Pork Steaks (page 114).
- Special Chicken and Black Bean Stir-fry (page 116).
- Basil Chicken (page 117).
- Chicken Bake (page 118).
- Chicken Casserole (page 119).
- Chicken and Mushroom Pasta (page 120).
- Chicken with Mushrooms (page 121).
- Chicken Paprika (page 122).
- Chicken and Sweetcorn Roll (page 123).

- Chicken Tikka (page 124).
- Jambalaya (page 125).
- Mediterranean Chicken (page 126).
- Pineapple and Cranberry Chicken (page 127).
- Sticky Ginger Chicken (page 128).
- Surprise, Surprise Chicken (page 129).
- Seasoned Chicken Portions (page 130).
- Stuffed Chicken Breasts (page 131).
- Tasty Citrus Chicken Parcels (page 133).
- Spicy Chicken or Turkey Burgers (page 134).
- Apricot Turkey Beanfeast (page 135).
- Exotic Turkey (page 136).
- Grilled Breast of Turkey in Basil and Mushroom Sauce (page 137).
- Turkey Bake (page 138).
- Turkey Bolognese (page 139).

Gourmet main courses: fish

- Cod in Mustard Sauce (page 140).
- Cod with Wine (page 141).
- Pasta Twirls with Scallops and Bacon (page 142).
- Poached Salmon with Dill Sauce (page 143).
- Quick and Easy Salmon with Dill (page 144).
- Salmon Olives in Asparagus Sauce (page 145).
- Special Fish Stir-fry (page 146).
- Haddock and Tomato Hotpot (page 152).
- Tuna Curry (page 151).
- Tuna Pasta (page 147).
- Tuna Chilli Tacos (page 149).
- Tuna Risotto (page 148).
- Tuna Quiche (page 150).

Gourmet main courses: vegetarian

- Cheesy Bean and Swede Layer (page 153).
- Chinese Vegetable Stir-fry (page 154).
- Continental Lentil Curry (page 155).
- Couscous Salad (page 156).
- Garlicky Stuffing and Lentil Layer (page 157).
- Lentil and Potato Pie (page 158).
- Pitta Cassoulet (page 159).
- Quick Pasta in Creamy Tomato and Mushroom Sauce (page 160).
- Quorn Pieces in French White Wine and Dill Sauce (page 161).
- Stir-fry Quorn (page 161).
- Vegetable Goulash (page 162).
- Vegetable Winter Bake (page 163).
- Vegetarian Chilli (page 164).
- Vegetable and Couscous Bake (page 165).
- Bean Soup (page 80).
- Red Lentil Soup (page 81).

Side dishes

- Fat-free Fluffy Rice (page 166).
- Dry-roast Potatoes (page 167).
- Garlic Potatoes (page 167).
- Dry-fried Mushrooms (page 168).
- Broad Bean and Mint Salad (page 168).
- Fire 'n' Ice Salad (page 169).
- Pinto Bean Salad (page 170).

Desserts

Select any one.

Quick and easy desserts

- 75g (3oz) fresh pineapple rings, topped with 1 liqueur glass of kirsch (optional) and 50g (2oz) pineapple-flavoured low-fat fromage frais.
- 115g (4oz) any fresh fruit, served with Banana and Creamy Topping (page 190).
- 2 brown Ryvitas spread with Marmite and topped with 50g (2oz) low-fat cottage cheese.
- 2 pieces any fresh fruit.
- 1 Boots Shapers Strawberry Fruit Sundae.
- 1 Boots Shapers Milk Chocolate Mousse.
- 1 x 100g serving Sainsbury's Apricot Halves in Apple Juice, topped with 1 apricot-flavoured diet yogurt or low-fat fromage frais containing no more than 50 calories.
- 1 x 100g serving Sainsbury's Fruit Cocktail in Grape Juice, topped with 1 diet yogurt or low-fat fromage frais containing no more than 50 calories.
- 1 x 150g serving St Michael Frozen Summer Fruits, plus 1 x 100g pot Boots Shapers Apricot Yoghurt Mousse.
- 1 x 100g serving St Michael Exotic Fruit Salad, plus 1 tablespoon low-fat fromage frais.
- 1 x 100g serving St Michael Sliced Mango in Syrup, plus 1 teaspoon low-fat fromage frais.

- 1 x 95g pot St Michael Summer Fruit Pudding.
- 2 x 100g pots St Michael Lite Fromage Frais.
- 1 x 100g pot St Michael Lite Fromage Frais, plus 1 piece fresh fruit.
- 1 x 100g serving St Michael Fruit Cocktail prepared in Light Syrup, plus 1 x 125g pot St Michael Very Low Fat Lite Yoghurt.
- 1 x 100g pot St Michael Fresh Oranges in Caramel with Grand Marnier Liqueur.
- 1 x St Michael Lite Mousse, any flavour.
- 1 x 150g pot St Michael Very Low Fat Lite Yoghurt, plus 115g (4oz) strawberries.
- 1 St Michael Very Low Fat Lite Yoghurt and Fruit twinpot.
- 1 x 100g pot St Michael Lite Natural Fromage Frais, plus 1 x 100g serving St Michael Red Fruit Summer Fruits Compote.
- 1 St Michael Luxury Meringue Nest, filled with either 1 tablespoon St Michael Lite Fromage Frais and 1 tablespoon St Michael Summer Fruits Compote or 115g (4oz) fresh fruit of your choice.
- 1 x 100ml serving Wall's 'Too Good To Be True' Total Toffee Temptation frozen dessert.
- 1 x 100ml serving Wall's 'Too Good To Be True' Vanilla frozen dessert.
- 1 x 100ml serving Wall's 'Too Good To Be True' Strawberry frozen dessert.
- 1 x 50ml serving Wall's 'Too Good To Be True' Strawberry frozen dessert, plus 115g (4oz) strawberries.
- 1 Weight Watchers from Heinz Low Fat Chocolate Mousse, plus 1 apple.

- 1 Weight Watchers from Heinz Yoplait Fat Free Fruit Yogurt, plus 1 piece fruit.
- 1 x 125ml or 61g serving Weight Watchers from Heinz Raspberry Whirl.
- 1 x 125ml or 61g serving Weight Watchers from Heinz Chocolate Swirl.
- 1 x 125ml or 61g serving Weight Watchers from Heinz Vanilla Iced Dessert.
- 1 x ⅙th serving Weight Watchers from Heinz Lemon Torte (380g pack).
- 1 x ⅕th serving Weight Watchers from Heinz Blackcurrant Torte (380g pack).
- 1 x 100ml serving Weight Watchers from Heinz Vanilla and Chocolate Chip Dolcetta.

Gourmet desserts

- Low-fat Chocolate Surprise Pudding (page 172).
- Crunchy Plum Crumble (page 173).
- Honey and Spice Pudding (page 173).
- Cranberry Pumpkin (page 174).
- Meringue Delight (page 175).
- Coffee and Banana Meringue (page 175).
- Low-fat Fruity Bread Pudding (page 176).
- Rhubarb and Blackcurrant Jelly (page 177).
- Rhubarb Jelly (page 177).
- Chocolate Mousse (page 178).
- Raspberry Mousse (page 178).
- Mango and Yogurt Mousse (page 179).
- Mango Sorbet (page 180).
- Chestnut Sundae (page 181).
- Morello Cherries and Melon Balls (page 182).

Snacks

Mid-morning and supper snacks

Select two items from this list per day. These are in addition to one snack taken from the mid-afternoon snacks list.

- 1 piece fresh fruit.
- 225g (8oz) melon excluding skin.
- 115g (4oz) fruit salad.
- 1 x 155g pack St Michael Fresh Melon Medley.
- Small salad made up of any salad vegetables, plus 1 tablespoon fat-free dressing.
- 1 sachet instant soup.
- 1 can Weight Watchers from Heinz Mediterranean Vegetable and Tomato Soup.
- 1 x 150g serving St Michael Pea and Mint Fresh Soup.
- 50g (2oz) low-fat cottage cheese, any flavour.
- 15g (½oz) cereal with milk from allowance.

- 9 Jacobs Iced Gems Mini Biscuits.
- 2 Jaffa Cakes.
- ½ packet polos or wine gums.
- 100ml (3fl oz) fresh orange juice.
- 1 tablespoon Wall's 'Too Good To Be True' frozen dessert.
- 1 x 50ml serving Weight Watchers from Heinz Vanilla and Chocolate Chip Dolcetta.
- 1 x 100g pot Weight Watchers from Heinz Fat Free Fromage Frais.
- 1 x 120g pot Weight Watchers from Heinz Fat Free Fruit Yogurt.
- 1 Weight Watchers from Heinz Low Fat Chocolate Mousse.
- 1 x 100g pot St Michael Lite Fromage Frais.
- 1 x 135g pack St Michael Summer Fruit Cocktail.
- 150g St Michael Frozen Bramley Apple and Blackberry.
- 115g (4oz) St Michael Frozen Tropical Fruits.
- 1 x 150g serving St Michael Frozen Summer Fruits.
- 50g (2oz) additional potatoes.
- 15g (½oz) [dry weight] additional rice.
- 15g (½oz) [dry weight] additional pasta.
- 25g (1oz) ham, chicken, or pastrami.
- 2 teaspoons sugar.
- 120ml (4fl oz) semi-skimmed milk in addition to allowance.
- 1 slice light bread.
- Crudités (chopped raw vegetables) with 75g (3oz) low-fat yogurt dip.
- 1 x 200g pack St Michael Carrot, Cauliflower and Broccoli Florets, eaten raw or microwaved.

Mid-afternoon snacks

Select one per day in addition to your mid-morning and supper snacks.

- 2 pieces fresh fruit.
- 1 slice light bread, toasted, plus 1 teaspoon marmalade.
- 1 slice light bread spread with mustard and topped with 15g (½oz) wafer thin ham, pork, beef, chicken or turkey, plus salad vegetables.
- Large salad made from selection of salad vegetables and 2 tablespoons low-fat salad dressing of your choice.
- 1 alcoholic drink in addition to allowance (maximum 3 per week).
- 25g (1oz) [dry weight] additional rice or pasta.
- 115g (4oz) additional potatoes.
- 1 slice light bread and 50g (2oz) baked beans.
- 1 St Michael Pikelet spread with 1 teaspoon jam and 1 teaspoon St Michael Lite Natural Fromage Frais.
- ½ x 400g (14oz) can regular soup.
- 1 can Weight Watchers from Heinz Carrot and Lentil Soup.
- 1 x 300g serving St Michael Pea and Mint Fresh Soup.
- 1 x ¼ serving St Michael Lite Fresh Vegetable Pizza.
- 1 piece fresh fruit, plus 1 low-fat fromage frais or yogurt containing no more than 50 calories.
- 1 Boots Shapers Strawberry Fruit Sundae.
- 1 Boots Shapers Yogurt Mousse, any flavour.

- 1 pack Boots Shapers American Style Bar-B-Cue Potato Waffles.
- 1 McVities Go Ahead Sticky Syrup and Fruit Cake Bar.
- 1 x 150g pot St Michael Low Fat Bio Yoghurt.
- 1 x 200g pot St Michael Extremely Fruity Low Fat Bio Yoghurt.
- 1 x 150g pot St Michael Very Low Fat Lite Yoghurt, plus wedge of melon.
- 1 x 100g pack St Michael Autumn Fruit Salad, plus 1 tablespoon St Michael Lite Natural Fromage Frais.
- 1 St Michael Lite Mousse, any flavour, plus 115g (4oz) strawberries.
- 1 x 100ml serving Weight Watchers from Heinz Vanilla and Choc Chip Dolcetta.
- 1 x ⅙th serving Weight Watchers from Heinz Lemon Torte (380g pack).
- 300ml (½ pint) Cool and Refreshing Yogurt Drink (page 191).
- 1 serving Not Naughty But Nice Strawberry Whip (page 190).
- 1 Strawberry Muffin (page 191).
- 1 slice Apple and Sultana Cake (page 192).
- 1 slice Spicy Apple Cake (page 192).
- 1 slice Coffee and Orange Slab (page 193).
- 1 slice Malt Loaf (page 194).

6
Recipes

Soup lunches
Salad lunches
Meat, poultry and fish lunches
Vegetarian lunches

Meat and poultry main courses
Fish main courses
Vegetarian main courses

Side dishes
Dressings
Desserts

Snacks

Soup Lunches

Bean Soup

SERVES 6

1 onion, chopped
1 teaspoon celery seed
1 teaspoon olive oil
½ cup canned flageolet beans
½ cup canned sweetcorn
1 carrot, chopped into small cubes
3 celery sticks, chopped into small cubes
1 potato, chopped into small cubes
1.2 litres (2 pints) vegetable stock
½ teaspoon dried basil or 1 teaspoon fresh basil
¼ teaspoon dried thyme or
½ teaspoon chopped fresh thyme
2 tablespoons chopped fresh parsley
salt and black pepper
skimmed milk from allowance (optional)

Sauté the onion and celery seed in the olive oil.

Place the onion and celery seed in a large pan. Add the beans, vegetables, vegetable stock, basil and thyme. Add 1 tablespoon of parsley and reserve the remainder for garnishing. Add salt and pepper to taste.

Cook until the vegetables are tender. Check the seasoning and adjust if necessary. A little skimmed milk can be added to thin the soup if required.

Just before serving, sprinkle the remaining parsley over. Serve hot, with 1 slice (40g/1½oz) wholemeal bread per person. (See note opposite.)

Red Lentil Soup

SERVES 4–6

175g (6oz) red lentils, rinsed
115g (4oz) leeks, sliced
75g (3oz) celery, sliced
1 litre (1¾ pints) vegetable stock
¼–½ teaspoon cayenne pepper (optional)
salt
4–6 tablespoons low-fat natural yogurt

Place the lentils, leeks, celery and stock in a large pan. Bring to the boil and simmer for about 25 minutes until the lentils are tender.

Allow the soup to cool a little, then transfer to a food processor or blender (or use a vegetable mill or a potato masher) and liquidise until smooth. Return to the pan and check the seasoning. Add the cayenne pepper (if using) a little at a time until the soup is to your taste. Add salt to taste if necessary.

Reheat the soup, adding a little more stock or water if necessary to give the consistency you like. Serve with a tablespoonful of yogurt on top of each dish and 1 slice (40g/1½oz) of wholemeal bread per person.

You may find this soup thickens considerably if left overnight (in the refrigerator). If it does, add more stock or water when you reheat it.

Note This soup and Bean Soup are also suitable as vegetarian main course options for dinner. Allow half the total recipe quantity per person and serve with 1 slice (40g/1½oz) wholemeal bread.

Vegetable Soup

SERVES 6

115g (4oz) onion
115g (4oz) celery
1 medium potato
½ teaspoon olive oil
¼ teaspoon dried thyme or
½ teaspoon chopped fresh thyme
1 bay leaf
salt and black pepper
1.2 litres (2 pints) chicken or vegetable stock

Peel, wash and roughly chop the vegetables.

Brush the bottom of large saucepan with a little olive oil. Add the vegetables, herbs, salt and black pepper. Place a lid on the pan and cook gently for about 5–10 minutes.

Add the stock, bring to boil and simmer for 15–20 minutes.

Transfer to a food processor or blender (or use a vegetable mill or a potato masher) and liquidise until smooth or until it is the consistency you prefer. Reheat, and serve with 1 slice (40g/1½oz) wholemeal bread per person, or separate into individual portions and freeze.

Variation Add one of the following to adapt the soup to your personal taste:

extra 115g (4oz) celery
extra 115g (4oz) onion
225g (8oz) cauliflower
225g (8oz) leeks
225g (8oz) carrots.

Salad Lunches

Prawn Salad

SERVES 1

75g (3oz) mixed salad leaves
1 large tomato, chopped
3 radishes, sliced
½ bunch watercress
75g (3oz) baby button mushrooms
115g (4oz) shelled prawns
75g (3oz) low-fat yogurt
1 tablespoon lemon juice
chopped fresh mint and parsley
salt and black pepper to taste

Place the salad leaves, tomato, radishes, mushrooms and prawns in a bowl and mix well.

Mix the yogurt with the lemon juice, mint and parsley and season to taste with the salt and black pepper. Pour over the salad ingredients and toss gently.

Serve immediately with 1 x 25g (1oz) bread roll.

Prawn and Mango Salad

SERVES 4

1 large ripe mango
½ sweet red pepper
½ sweet yellow pepper
1 lime
½–1 teaspoon finely chopped green or red chilli
(remove the seeds if you do not want
the dressing to be too hot)
2 tablespoons chopped fresh coriander or parsley
2 tablespoons low-fat natural yogurt or fromage frais
225g (8oz) peeled prawns
mixed salad leaves

Peel the mango, remove the stone and chop the flesh finely.

Grate the rind of the lime finely and squeeze the juice from the lime. Deseed the peppers, dice finely and place in a bowl. Add the mango, lime juice and rind, chopped chilli, coriander or parsley and the prawns. Mix gently together, cover and refrigerate for 2 hours.

To make the dressing, drain the liquid from the mixture into a bowl and stir the yogurt or fromage frais into the liquid. Mix well.

Place the mixed salad leaves in the base of 4 glasses and, just before serving, spoon the prawn and mango mixture into each glass and pour some of the dressing over each.

Variation As an alternative you could substitute fresh tomatoes (peeled, seeded and diced) for the mango and use a dash of Tabasco sauce instead of the chilli.

Sardine, Beetroot and Red Apple Salad

SERVES 2

1 x 120g (4.2oz) can sardines in brine
50g (2oz) low-fat natural yogurt
75g (3oz) cooked and grated beetroot
1 red apple, grated (leave skin on)
pepper to taste
1 small lettuce

Drain and mash the sardines. Mix in the yogurt, stir in the beetroot and apple and season well.

Chill and serve on a bed of lettuce.

Kipper Salad

SERVES 1

1 x 75g (3oz) kipper fillet
1 medium orange
25g (1oz) cooked rice
175g (6oz) mixed cucumber,
tomato and green pepper, chopped
4 teaspoons low-fat salad dressing

Skin the kipper fillet and poach the fish in water. Drain well, then flake coarsely.

Cut the peel from the orange and cut out the segments with a small sharp knife. Squeeze any juice from the remainder of the orange. Mix the kipper fillet with the rice and chopped vegetables. Add the salad dressing and any juice from the orange and mix well.

Pile into a dish and garnish with the orange slices.

Crispy Vegetable Salad

SERVES 4

450g (1lb) small new potatoes
unlimited quantities of mange-tout
and baby sweetcorn
1 bunch spring onions
1 carton Asda 95% Fat Free Onion and Garlic Dip
1 lettuce

Scrub the potatoes and cook in boiling salted water until tender. Drain them, then place under cold running water until completely cold. Drain well.

Blanch the mange-tout and baby sweetcorn in boiling salted water for 2 minutes. Drain and chill in the same way as the potatoes.

Trim and finely slice the spring onions. Dice the potatoes and cut the mange-tout and sweetcorn in half or into short lengths. Mix all the vegetables together with the onion and garlic dip.

Wash the lettuce and arrange the leaves in a large bowl or on individual plates and pile the vegetable mixture in the centre.

Variation If you wish to make your own onion and garlic dip, crush one or two cloves of garlic into a 450g (1lb) carton of low-fat cottage cheese or fromage frais. If you prefer a stronger flavour of onion, grate half a medium onion into the cottage cheese or fromage frais.

Fruit and Chicken Salad

SERVES 1

unlimited amounts of shredded lettuce,
chopped cucumber and any other green salad
1 apple
1 pear
1 orange
1 kiwi fruit
50g (2oz) cooked chicken breast, chopped

for the dressing
2 tablespoons low-fat natural yogurt
1 tablespoon wine vinegar
1 garlic clove, peeled and crushed
salt and freshly ground black pepper

Place the lettuce and green salad on a large dinner plate.

Prepare the fruits by peeling, coring and slicing. Lay the slices in a circle on top of the salad vegetables and place the chopped chicken in the centre.

Mix together the dressing ingredients, and pour over the salad.

Meat, Poultry and Fish Lunches

Crispy Topped Mushrooms

SERVES 4

Vegetarians can adapt this recipe by omitting the bacon and adding an extra 25g (1oz) low-fat cheese.

4 large open mushrooms
1 small onion, chopped
4 lean back rashers bacon, chopped
1 x 200g (7oz) can chopped tomatoes
1 teaspoon Worcester sauce
1 teaspoon soy sauce
salt and pepper
$\frac{1}{4}$–$\frac{1}{2}$ teaspoon sugar

for the topping
4 tablespoons fresh breadcrumbs
25g (1oz) grated low-fat cheese
$\frac{1}{2}$–1 teaspoon mixed herbs

Peel the mushrooms and remove the stalks. Put the mushrooms to one side and chop the stalks.

Dry-fry the mushroom stalks, chopped onion and bacon for 5 minutes, then add the tomatoes, Worcester sauce and soy sauce. Season to taste with salt and pepper and sugar. Simmer gently until the mixture is thick.

Place the reserved mushrooms in a large frying pan with a little water. Cook until they are almost tender and liquid has been absorbed. Remove from the heat. Fill the mushrooms with the tomato and bacon mixture.

To make the topping, mix the breadcrumbs, low-fat cheese and mixed herbs and sprinkle over each mushroom. Cook under a hot grill until brown and crispy.

Serve with a salad or green vegetables.

Banana Surprise

SERVES 4

4 bananas
a little cinnamon
1 x 150g (5oz) pack turkey rashers
chutney (optional)

Sprinkle the bananas with a little cinnamon and wrap a turkey rasher around each one. Wrap each one in foil, place on a baking sheet and cook in a preheated oven at 200C, 400F or Gas Mark 6 for 15–20 minutes until the bacon and bananas are cooked. Alternatively, you can cook them (without the foil) over a hot barbeque for 15 minutes.

Unwrap the foil parcels and serve the bananas with a little chutney if you wish and a mixed salad.

Savoury Cauliflower Bake

SERVES 2

Vegetarians can adapt this recipe by omitting the bacon, substituting mushroom soup for the chicken soup and sprinkling 25g (1oz) grated low-fat cheese over the top.

1 medium cauliflower
salt
25g (1oz) lean back bacon, chopped
1 medium onion, chopped
115g (4oz) mushrooms, chopped
1 x 295g can low-calorie chicken soup
4 tablespoons low-fat natural yogurt

Break the cauliflower into florets, rinse and cook in boiling salted water. Drain and place in an ovenproof dish.

Dry-fry the bacon, onion and mushrooms, then place on top of the cauliflower.

Mix the soup with the yogurt and pour over the caulifower mixture. Bake in a preheated oven at 200C, 400F or Gas Mark 6 for 30 minutes, or microwave on High for 3–4 minutes then brown under the grill.

Turkey Rashers with Chilli and Pasta

SERVES 4

1 x 150g (5oz) pack turkey rashers, cut into pieces
1 onion, chopped
1 green chilli, chopped, or chilli powder to taste
1 x 400g (14oz) can chopped tomatoes
salt
175g (6oz) [dry weight] pasta shells

Dry-fry the onion and turkey rashers until lightly browned. Add the chilli and the tomatoes and season to taste with salt. Bring to the boil and simmer for 10–15 minutes until the sauce has thickened slightly.

In the meantime, cook the pasta in boiling salted water. When cooked, drain well and add to the turkey mixture. Stir thoroughly so that the pasta is coated. Check the seasoning and serve immediately with a green salad.

Pasta with Spinach Sauce

SERVES 2

Vegetarians can use this recipe and omit the anchovies.

50g (2oz) [dry weight] wholewheat fusilli pasta
300g (12oz) fresh spinach or
150g (6oz) frozen spinach
115g (4oz) quark
salt and black pepper
a little low-fat fromage frais or skimmed milk
50g (2oz) can fillets of anchovies

Cook the pasta as directed and drain well.

Wash the fresh spinach (if using) and cook in 1 tablespoon of water. Drain well and chop finely in a food processor or with a knife. If using frozen spinach, cook as directed.

Mix the quark with the spinach, and add salt and pepper to taste. If the mixture is too stiff, add a little low-fat fromage frais or skimmed milk.

Drain the anchovies and wash well to remove the oil from the surface. Pat dry on kitchen paper, then chop.

Heat the spinach sauce, add the cooked pasta and pile onto serving plates. Top with the anchovies and serve with a green salad and crusty French bread (50g/2oz per person).

Tuna Burgers

SERVES 4

350g (12oz) old potatoes
1 x 185g (6½oz) can tuna in water or
brine, drained and flaked
115g (4oz) canned sweetcorn, drained
2 tablespoons chopped fresh parsley
salt and black pepper
1 tablespoon flour

Peel the potatoes and boil in salted water for 20 minutes or until tender. Drain then mash them and leave to cool for 5 minutes. When cool, add the tuna, sweetcorn and parsley and season to taste. Mix well again. Transfer the mixture onto a floured board. Divide the mixture into 4 and shape into burgers.

Dry-fry the tuna burgers in a non-stick pan over a medium heat for 5–7 minutes, turning them occasionally, until they are heated through. Alternatively, cook under a medium hot grill for 7–10 minutes, turning them once.

Serve with baked beans or unlimited salad.

Tuna Fish Pie

SERVES 4

450g (1lb) potatoes
salt
1 x 400g (14oz) can tuna in brine
1 x 295g (11oz) can Campbell's
Condensed Half Fat Mushroom Soup
2–3 pickled onions

Cook the potatoes in boiling salted water, then drain and mash them.

Drain the tuna and place in the bottom of an oven-proof dish. Pour the soup over.

Chop the onions and sprinkle over the tuna. Spread the mashed potatoes on top and bake in a preheated oven at 190C, 375F or Gas Mark 5 for 30–40 minutes until brown.

Serve with unlimited salad.

Vegetarian Lunches

Courgette Provençale

SERVES 4

6 courgettes, sliced
2 onions, chopped
1 x 400g (14oz) chopped tomatoes
1 teaspoon garlic purée
50g (2oz) vegetarian cheese

Place the courgettes and onions in an ovenproof dish.

Mash the tomatoes and garlic purée in a bowl. Pour over the courgettes and onions. Sprinkle the cheese on top.

Bake in a preheated oven at 200C, 400F or Gas Mark 6 for 20 minutes.

Serve with a selection of additional vegetables and either boiled pasta (50g/2oz dry weight per person) or 175g (6oz) potatoes.

Tomato and Cheese Tarts

SERVES 4

2 sheets filo pastry
1 egg white
350g (12oz) low-fat cottage cheese
handful of fresh basil leaves
3 tomatoes, sliced
salt and black pepper

Brush the sheets of filo pastry lightly with the egg white and cut into 16 x 10cm (4 inch) squares.

Place the squares in layers of twos in 8 patty tins, so that the 2 squares criss-cross to form an angle to each other. Spoon the cheese on top of the squares, sprinkle with pepper and top with basil.

Arrange the tomato slices on top and sprinkle with salt.

Bake in a preheated oven at 200C, 400F or Gas Mark 6 for 10–12 minutes.

Serve warm.

Red Kidney Bean Curry

SERVES 4

2 onions, chopped
1 x 2.5cm (1 inch) stick cinnamon
2 garlic cloves, chopped
1 red pepper, sliced
1 green pepper, sliced
½ teaspoon chilli powder
1½ teaspoons ground coriander
1 teaspoon ground cumin
1 teaspoon garam masala
¼ teaspoon turmeric
1 x 400g (14oz) can chopped tomatoes
salt to taste
1 x 400g (14oz) can kidney beans, drained

Dry-fry the onions in a large non-stick pan until soft. Add the cinnamon, garlic and peppers and fry for 1 minute. Add the chilli powder, coriander, cumin, garam masala and turmeric, stirring all the time. Add the tomatoes and season to taste with salt. Cover and simmer for 5 minutes.

Add the kidney beans and a little water if required and simmer for a further 5 minutes.

Serve with boiled brown rice (allow 50g/2oz dry weight per person) or 1 large pitta bread.

Creamy Cauliflower Pasta

SERVES 2

1 large onion, chopped
2 garlic cloves, crushed
1 small cauliflower, broken into florets
115g (4oz) button mushrooms
1 x 295g (11oz) can Campbell's
Condensed Half Fat Mushroom Soup
skimmed milk from allowance
salt and pepper
50g (2oz) grated low-fat Cheddar cheese

Dry-fry the onion and garlic in a non-stick pan.

Add just a little water to the pan, then add the cauliflower florets. Place a lid on the pan and simmer until the cauliflower is tender. Add the mushrooms to the pan and cook for 1 minute.

Pour the soup into the pan. Use the empty can to measure the milk. Pour the milk into the can until the can is approximately three-quarters full, then add to the pan. Season to taste. Heat through gently until bubbling.

Place in a heatproof dish and sprinkle the grated cheese over the top. Place under the grill to brown.

Serve with cooked pasta shells (allow 50g/2oz dry weight per person).

Variation Use asparagus soup instead of mushroom soup and substitute a can of asparagus spears for the mushrooms. Cut the spears into small pieces and add at the same time as the soup.

Ratatouille au Gratin

SERVES 1–2

1 courgette, sliced
1 aubergine, sliced
1 x 400g (14oz) can chopped tomatoes
½ x 200g (7oz) can sweetcorn, drained
115g (4oz) mushrooms
25g (1oz) chilli sauce
1 slice brown bread, grated
25–50g (1–2oz) grated low-fat cheese

Place all the vegetables and the chilli sauce in an ovenproof dish. Mix the bread and cheese and sprinkle on top.

Bake in a preheated oven at 190C, 375F or Gas Mark 5 for 30 minutes to 1 hour until crisp and bubbling.

Baked Artichokes with Apricots

SERVES 2–3

1 x 425g (15oz) can artichoke hearts, drained
225g (8oz) low-fat cottage cheese
225g (8oz) low-fat fromage frais
2 fresh apricots
salt and pepper

Place the drained artichoke hearts in an ovenproof dish.

Combine the fromage frais and cottage cheese.

Peel, core and finely chop the apricots and mix well with the cheese mixture. Pour over the artichoke hearts and season lightly with salt and pepper.

Cover and bake in a preheated oven at 180C, 350F, or Gas Mark 4 for 15 minutes.

Serve with salad.

Creamy Curried Quorn

SERVES 2

1 vegetable stock cube
225g (8oz) Quorn chunks
3 tablespoons Kraft Fat Free Yoghurt and
Chive Dressing
1 teaspoon curry powder
50g (2oz) [dry weight] brown rice
1 tablespoon chopped fresh parsley to garnish

Dissolve the stock cube in boiling water. Simmer the Quorn in vegetable stock for 15–20 minutes. Drain and allow to cool.

Mix together the dressing and curry powder and add to the Quorn. Leave overnight in the refrigerator for the flavours to develop.

Cook the rice according to the instructions. Drain well and leave to cool.

Garnish the Quorn with the chopped parsley and serve chilled on a bed of rice. Serve with a mixed salad.

Toasted Muffin Pizza

SERVES 1

1 wholemeal muffin
115g (4oz) low-fat cottage cheese
2 teaspoons tomato purée or tomato sauce
mixed herbs to taste

Cut the muffin in half and toast the outside under a grill. Turn over and spread the other side with the tomato purée or sauce. Top with the cottage cheese, and sprinkle the mixed herbs on top. Place under the grill to brown.

Serve with salad.

Pepper and Wholewheat Pasta

SERVES 3–4

175g (6oz) wholewheat pasta shells
175g (6oz) broccoli florets
salt
1 onion, sliced
1 garlic clove, crushed
1 yellow pepper and 1 red pepper, sliced
2 courgettes
1 tablespoon brown sugar
2 tomatoes, quartered
1 tablespoon white wine vinegar
chopped fresh basil to garnish

Cook the pasta according to the instructions.

Blanch the broccoli in boiling salted water and drain well.

Dry-fry the onion and garlic in a non-stick pan until the onion is transparent. Add the peppers and courgettes and cook for a further 2 minutes. Add the broccoli and the brown sugar and cook for a further 2 minutes.

When the pasta is cooked, drain well and place in a serving dish. Mix the tomatoes and white wine vinegar with the pasta. Add the other ingredients and mix well.

Garnish with fresh basil and serve cold.

Meat and Poultry Main Courses

Lamb Burgers

SERVES 4

450g (1lb) lean minced lamb
1 small onion, finely chopped
2 tablespoons tomato ketchup
salt and pepper

Mix all the ingredients together and season well with salt and pepper.

Divide the mixture into 4 portions and shape into burgers.
Cook each burger under a very hot grill or on a barbecue for 5–6 minutes on each side.

Serve with 175g (6oz) potatoes or a wholemeal bap per person, plus unlimited vegetables of your choice.

Lamb and Pineapple Curry

SERVES 4

If you prefer a mild curry, use less curry powder or a milder one.

1 large onion, sliced
1 garlic clove, crushed
1 tablespoon plain flour
1–2 tablespoons Madras curry powder
350g (12oz) lean lamb, cubed
1 tablespoon tomato purée
600ml (1 pint) beef stock
115g (4oz) pineapple cubes canned in natural juice
salt and pepper

Dry-fry the onion and garlic in a non-stick pan until soft. Place in a casserole dish.

Mix the flour and curry powder together. Toss the lamb in this mixture, then dry-fry until brown. Place in the casserole dish.

Stir the remaining flour and curry mixture into the hot pan and cook for a moment or two. Stir in the tomato purée and a little stock. Stir well to loosen any mixture from the base of the pan. Gradually add the rest of the stock, stirring occasionally, and bring to the boil. Pour the sauce over the lamb. Stir the pineapple cubes into the lamb curry and season to taste.

Cover and cook in a preheated oven at 180C, 350F or Gas Mark 4 for 1 hour or until the lamb is tender.

Check the seasoning and serve with boiled rice (allow 25g/1oz dry weight per person) plus unlimited vegetables.

Savoury Lamb Mince

SERVES 4

450g (1lb) lean lamb mince
1 medium onion, chopped
1 teaspoon garlic paste
1 teaspoon red chilli powder
½ teaspoon turmeric
1 x 400g (14oz) can chopped tomatoes
1 tablespoon tomato purée
salt and pepper

Dry-fry the mince in a heavy-based pan until brown. Drain through a colander or sieve to remove any fat, then spread the mince on kitchen paper. Pat gently to absorb as much fat as possible. Wipe out the pan.

Dry-fry the onion for about 3–4 minutes until it starts to soften. Add the garlic paste, red chilli powder and turmeric and mix well.

Return the mince to the pan. Add the tomatoes and the tomato purée. Season to taste. Mix well and continue to cook over a low heat for a further 20 minutes or until the meat is tender.

Serve with boiled rice (allow 25g/1oz dry weight per person) or 175g (6oz) potatoes per person and unlimited vegetables of your choice.

Faggots with Gravy

SERVES 2

175g (6oz) lamb's or pork liver
1 teaspoon dried onion flakes or
1 small onion, finely chopped
3 tablespoons fresh breadcrumbs
¼ teaspoon mixed herbs
2–3 teaspoons low-fat onion or
beef instant gravy granules

Place the liver in a pan. Pour about 300ml (½ pint) boiling water over. Bring to the boil, turn off the heat and leave for 2 minutes.

Remove the liver from the pan and reserve the cooking liquor.

Mince the liver together with the onion flakes or onion in a food processor or mincer. Stir in the breadcrumbs and mixed herbs and season lightly.

Form the mixture into 4 balls and place in an ovenproof dish. Pour 2–3 tablespoons of the cooking liquor into the dish and bake in a preheated oven at 190C, 375F or Gas Mark 5 for about 20 minutes until lightly browned.

Make the remaining cooking liquor up to 250ml (8fl oz) with water. Bring to the boil and make the gravy according to the instructions. Stir well.

Pour the gravy around the faggots and serve with unlimited vegetables of your choice.

Autumn Country Bake

SERVES 4

450g (1lb) lean minced beef
115g (4oz) mushrooms, sliced
1 medium onion, sliced
1 x 200g (7oz) can sweetcorn, drained
250ml (8fl oz) beef stock
1 teaspoon dried mixed herbs
450g (1lb) potatoes
salt

Dry-fry the mince in a non-stick pan or wok until brown. Remove the mince, drain off any excess fat through a colander or sieve and wipe the pan or wok.

Return the mince to the pan or wok, add the mushrooms and onion and cook for about 5 minutes, stirring occasionally.

Add the sweetcorn, beef stock and herbs and bring to the boil. Cover and simmer gently for 15 minutes.

In the meantime, cook the potatoes in boiling salted water. When cooked, drain well, then mash to a soft consistency using water or a little milk.

Transfer the meat mixture to an ovenproof dish. Top with the mashed potato and bake in a preheated oven at 190C, 375F or Gas Mark 5 for 30 minutes.

If necessary, brown under a hot grill for a couple of minutes.

Serve with unlimited vegetables.

Beef and Orange Curry

SERVES 4

This is a very hot curry. If you prefer a milder curry, use less curry powder or a milder one.

450g (1lb) lean braising steak, trimmed and
cut into 2cm (¾ inch) dice
1 medium onion, chopped
2 garlic cloves, crushed
1–2 tablespoons Madras curry powder
450ml (3/4 pint) beef stock
salt and pepper
4 medium oranges
2 teaspoons cornflour

Dry-fry the beef, onion and garlic in a heavy-based pan until brown.

Add the curry powder and cook for a further 1–2 minutes.

Add the stock, season to taste and bring to the boil. Lower the heat, cover and simmer gently for 1 hour or until the meat is tender.

In the meantime, grate the rind from one of the oranges and squeeze the juice from this and a second orange. Cut the peel and pith from the remaining two oranges and cut out the segments from each orange.

When the beef is tender, blend the cornflour with a little of the orange juice. Stir the blended cornflour, the grated orange rind and remaining juice into the curry. Bring to the boil, stirring continuously, and simmer for about 5 minutes until slightly thickened.

Check the seasoning and stir in the orange segments.

Serve with boiled rice (allow 25g/1oz dry weight per person), grilled pappads (1 per person) and cucumber raita made with 300ml (½ pint) low-fat yogurt mixed with 1 small chopped cucumber.

Mince and Ginger Stir-Fry

SERVES 4

1 x 2.5cm (1 inch) piece root ginger
3–4 garlic cloves
450 g (1lb) lean minced beef or turkey
4 pineapple rings canned in natural juice
1 green or red pepper
450g (1lb) broccoli or cauliflower or a mixture of both
2 tablespoons soy sauce or to taste
salt and pepper
150ml (¼ pint) stock (optional)

Peel the ginger and garlic and cut into very small pieces or grate coarsely.

Heat a heavy-based pan or wok. Add the ginger, garlic and the mince and cook for 10–15 minutes, stirring occasionally, until the mince is brown.

Dice the pineapple and cut the pepper into strips. Cut the broccoli and/or cauliflower into small florets. Add the pepper, the broccoli or cauliflower and the soy sauce to the pan. Season to taste with salt and pepper.

Cook over a gentle heat for a further 10–15 minutes until the vegetables are tender. Add a tablespoon or two of stock as necessary to give sufficient liquid for the vegetables to cook. Check the seasoning and serve with 115g (4oz) [cooked weight] boiled rice per person.

Bacon and Runner Bean Stir-Fry

SERVES 4

350g (12oz) lean bacon rashers
2 red, green or yellow peppers, thinly sliced
2 medium onions, thinly sliced
115g (4oz) mushrooms, sliced
225g (8oz) frozen runner beans

Remove all the fat from the bacon and discard. Cut the bacon into pieces. Place in a hot heavy-based pan or wok and cook until lightly browned, stirring occasionally.

Add the peppers, onions and mushrooms and cook for 5 minutes or until the vegetables are nearly tender.

Add the runner beans and season lightly. Continue cooking, stirring occasionally, until all the water from the beans has evaporated.

Check the seasoning and serve with 175g (6oz) jacket potatoes per person.

Italian-style Gammon Steaks

SERVES 4

This dish tastes even better cold the next day.

115–150g (4–5oz) [dry weight] pasta spirals
1 x 400g (14oz) can ratatouille
1 x 200g (7oz) can chopped tomatoes
1 small onion, finely chopped
1 Italian stock cube
4 x 115g (4 x 4oz) St Michael
Low Fat Gammon Steaks

Cook the pasta in boiling salted water until just tender. Drain well.

In the meantime, empty the can of ratatouille and the can of tomatoes into a pan. Add the chopped onion and stock cube and simmer for 8–10 minutes until the onion is tender.

While the sauce is cooking, dry-fry the gammon steaks until tender or, if you prefer, poach them in a little water.

Stir the cooked pasta into the sauce and pile into a serving dish. Arrange the gammon steaks on top and serve with a salad or unlimited vegetables.

Leek and Ham Cannelloni

SERVES 4

4 medium leeks, cut in half
1 x 295g (11oz) can Campbell's
Condensed Half Fat Mushroom Soup
8 x 50g (8 x 2oz) slices lean ham
2 slices wholemeal bread, made into breadcrumbs

Cook the leeks in boiling water until just tender. Drain well as they tend to hold a lot of water (if necessary place them on kitchen paper to dry).

Heat the soup with 150ml (1/4 pint) water.

Wrap a slice of ham around each leek half and place in an ovenproof dish. Pour the soup over so that all the leeks are covered. Sprinkle the breadcrumbs on top and bake in a preheated oven at 190C, 375F or Gas Mark 5 for about 20 minutes or until golden brown on top. Serve hot with 175g (6oz) jacket potatoes per person.

Savoury Rice with Ham

SERVES 1

Vegetarians can adapt this dish by omitting the ham and stirring 50g (2oz) low-fat grated cheese into the mixture after the liquid has been absorbed.

50g (2oz) onion, chopped
50g (2oz) mushrooms, chopped
1 teaspoon tomato purée
1 x 200g (7oz) can chopped tomatoes
dash of Worcester sauce
25g (1oz) [dry weight] rice
75g (3oz) lean cooked ham, diced

Dry-fry the onions and mushrooms in a non-stick pan. Add the tomato purée, tomatoes, Worcester sauce and the uncooked rice. Season lightly with salt and pepper, bring to the boil, cover and simmer gently until the rice is tender.

Add the ham to the pan, raise the heat and continue cooking, uncovered, until the liquid has been absorbed. Stir the mixture occasionally so that the rice does not stick to the bottom of the pan. Check the seasoning.

Serve hot with a salad.

Chinese Pork with Ginger

SERVES 3

350g (12oz) lean pork fillet
2 tablespoons oyster sauce
1 tablespoon soy sauce
2 tablespoons dry white wine or cider
1 tablespoon clear honey
1 x 5cm (2 inch) piece root ginger, peeled and grated

Thinly slice the pork.

Mix all the other ingredients together in a small bowl. Add the pork and stir until all the meat is coated with the sauce. Leave to marinate for 30 minutes.

Heat a heavy-based pan or wok. Remove the pork from the sauce and dry-fry for 4 minutes.

Add the sauce and cook for a further 3 minutes.

Serve with boiled noodles (allow 25g/1oz dry weight per person) and Chinese vegetables or vegetables of your choice.

Gingered Pork with Apricots

SERVES 4

450g (1lb) lean pork, cubed
1 medium onion, chopped
1 teaspoon dried ginger
1 teaspoon chopped fresh thyme
75g (3oz) ready-to-use dried apricots
600ml (1 pint) vegetable or pork stock
salt and pepper
2 teaspoons cornflour

Cook the pork and onion in a hot heavy-based pan on a hob, stirring occasionally, until the pork is browned.

Add the ginger, thyme, apricots and stock. Season to taste with salt and pepper and bring to the boil.

Mix the cornflour with a little cold water and stir into the pan, mixing well.

Pour the meat and sauce into a casserole dish. Cover and place in a preheated oven at 180C, 350F or Gas Mark 4. Cook for 1–1¼ hours until the pork is tender.

Check the seasoning. Serve with 175g (6oz) potatoes per person and unlimited vegetables.

Pork and Apple Parcels

SERVES 4

40g (1½oz) sage and onion stuffing mix
1 large onion, thinly sliced
300ml (½ pint) chicken stock
350g (12oz) small old potatoes, thinly sliced
1 large cooking apple, peeled and sliced
4 x 115g (4 x 4oz) pork chops or pork steaks
salt and freshly ground black pepper
2 teaspoons low-fat gravy granules (optional)

Mix the sage and onion stuffing mix with 150ml (¼ pint) boiling water and leave to stand for 10–15 minutes.

Cook the onion in the chicken stock for 6–7 minutes until almost tender. Remove the onion from the pan with a slotted spoon.

Place the potato slices in the stock and cook for 3–4 minutes until they are nearly soft. Carefully remove the potatoes from the pan with a slotted spoon and reserve any remaining stock to make the gravy if desired.

Take 4 large pieces of aluminium foil and place a quarter of the potatoes, onions and apples on each.

Remove all the fat from the pork chops or steaks. Dry-fry the pork in a non-stick pan for a few minutes until browned on both sides.

Place a pork chop or steak on each pile of vegetables and top with the stuffing mixture. Season with salt and pepper. Fold the foil over to seal the parcels well. Place on a baking tray and cook in a preheated oven at 200C, 400F or Gas Mark 6 for 25–30 minutes until the meat is tender.

Make up the gravy (if using) with the reserved stock and the gravy granules and pour into a gravy boat.

Place the pork parcels on a serving dish so that each person can open their own parcel.

Serve hot with green vegetables and gravy.

Pork Crumble

SERVES 4

450g (1lb) pork shoulder steaks,
cut into 8 medallions
1 x 376g (13¼oz) can Homepride Tomato and
Onion Sauce
75g (3oz) stuffing mix

Place the pork in an ovenproof dish and pour the sauce over. Sprinkle the dry stuffing mix over the top, pat it in and cover the dish with a tight-fitting lid or foil.

Place in a preheated oven at 190C, 375F or Gas Mark 5 for 40 minutes or until the pork is tender.

Serve with Dry-roast Potatoes (page 167) and unlimited fresh vegetables.

Pork Stroganoff

SERVES 4

350g (12oz) lean pork fillet or tenderloin
115g (4oz) lean bacon
1–2 tablespoons seasoned flour
115g (4oz) mushrooms
1 x 295g (11oz) can Campbell's Condensed
Half Fat Mushroom Soup
1 rounded tablespoon tomato purée
1 x 150g (5oz) low-fat natural yogurt
salt and pepper

Trim away any fat from the pork and bacon and discard. Cut the pork and bacon into thin strips.

Toss the pork in the seasoned flour.

Heat a heavy-based pan and dry-fry the pork until brown. Remove from the pan.

Slice the mushrooms. Add the mushrooms and bacon to the pan and cook lightly for a few minutes.

Return the pork to the pan, pour the soup into the pan and mix in the tomato purée and yogurt. Check the seasoning. Mix well together and bring to the boil. Cover and simmer slowly for 20 minutes or until the meat is tender.

Serve with 175g (6oz) jacket potatoes per person and vegetables of your choice, or boiled rice (allow 25g/1oz dry weight per person) and a crisp green salad.

Zingy Limed Pork Steaks

SERVES 4

4 x 115g (4 x 4oz) lean pork steaks
2 limes
1 medium onion, chopped
250ml (8fl oz) vegetable stock
15g (½oz) cornflour
1 tablespoon skimmed milk
2 tablespoons dry vermouth
salt and pepper
2 tablespoons low-fat fromage frais

Grill or barbecue the steaks for 8–10 minutes each side or until cooked through and tender.

In the meantime, cut 4 thin slices from one of the limes. Grate the rind from the remainder of this one and the second lime and squeeze out the juice from both. Reserve.

Make the sauce in either of the following ways:

Microwave

Place the onion in a microwave dish and cook on High for 2 minutes. Add the juice and rind from the limes. Add the onion and the vegetable stock then microwave for a further 3 minutes.

Slake the cornflour with the milk and add to the dish. Add the vermouth. Season to taste with salt and pepper and mix well.

Microwave for a further 30 seconds.

Leave to stand for 2 minutes, then stir in the fromage frais. Check the seasoning and serve.

Conventional method

Dry-fry the onion gently in a hot non-stick pan, stirring occasionally until the onion is translucent and only lightly coloured.

Add the grated rind and juice from the limes. Add the stock and cook until the onion is tender. If necessary, add a little more stock or water to maintain the original amount of liquid.

Slake the cornflour in the milk and add to the pan. Stir in the vermouth. Bring to the boil and simmer for 2–3 minutes.

Season to taste. Remove from the heat, stir in the fromage frais and reheat gently without boiling. Check the seasoning and serve.

To serve

Place the steaks on a hot serving dish, pour the sauce over and garnish with the reserved slices of lime.

Serve with 175g (6oz) new potatoes per person and calabrese or a mixed salad or unlimited vegetables.

Special Chicken and Black Bean Stir-fry

SERVES 2

1 x 115g (4oz) boned and skinned chicken breast,
cut into strips
50g (2oz) lean pork, cut into strips
150g (5oz) mixed peppers,
cut into 2.5cm (1 inch) pieces
5 tablespoons black bean sauce
75g (3oz) mushrooms, sliced
75g (3oz) cooked peeled prawns
2 tablespoons dry sherry
50g (2oz) [dry weight] white rice
salt and pepper

Pour boiling water over the chicken and pork and leave in the water for 5 minutes, then strain. Do the same with the peppers.

Heat a wok or heavy-based pan, add the black bean sauce and heat gently. Add the drained meat, the peppers and the mushrooms and cook gently in the sauce for 4–5 minutes or until the meat and peppers are tender.

Stir in the prawns and sherry and heat through.

In the meantime, boil the rice according to the instructions. Drain.

Check the seasoning of the sauce, pile the cooked rice onto a serving dish and pour the chicken mixture over.

Serve hot.

Basil Chicken

SERVES 4

4 x 115g (4 x 4oz) boned and
skinned chicken breasts
chopped fresh basil to taste
4 tablespoons fresh white breadcrumbs
salt and black pepper
a little skimmed milk
175–225g (6–8oz) fresh asparagus spears or
1 x 400g (14oz) can asparagus spears
to garnish (optional)

Slightly flatten the chicken breasts.

Add plenty of basil to the breadcrumbs so that the mixture smells strongly of the herb. Season with salt and lots of black pepper.

Dip the chicken breasts into the milk and coat with the breadcrumb and herb mixture.

Dry-fry the chicken in a non-stick pan for a few minutes until both sides are brown.

Place the chicken breasts on a non-stick baking tray and cook in a preheated oven at 180C, 350F or Gas Mark 4 for 15 minutes.

Garnish with asparagus spears if desired and serve with 175g (6oz) potatoes per person and unlimited vegetables of your choice.

Chicken Bake

SERVES 4

450g (1lb) new potatoes
1 medium onion, chopped
1 garlic clove, crushed (optional)
4 x 115–150g (4 x 4–5 oz) boned and
skinned chicken breasts
150–300 ml (¼–½ pint) chicken stock
225g (8oz) mushrooms, sliced
1 red pepper, sliced into rings
salt and pepper
mixed herbs to taste

Peel the potatoes if you wish and cook in boiling salted water until nearly tender. Drain well and cut into 5mm (¼ inch) slices.

Heat a non-stick or heavy-based pan, add the onion and garlic (if using) and dry-fry gently, stirring frequently, until the onion is lightly browned.

Remove the onion from the pan. Add the chicken breasts and dry-fry until brown on both sides.

Pour a little of the stock into the pan, add the mushrooms and red pepper and cook until just tender. Season lightly.

Arrange a layer of potato slices in the bottom of an ovenproof dish. Place the chicken breasts on top, followed by the vegetables. Sprinkle a few mixed herbs over and cover with the remaining potato slices.

Pour about 150ml (¼ pint) of stock over. Cover with a tight-fitting lid or foil and bake in a preheated oven at 180C, 350F or Gas Mark 4 for approximately 40 minutes.

Remove the lid and turn the oven up to 190C, 375F or Gas Mark 5 and cook for a further 10 minutes until the potato is golden, adding more stock if necessary to keep the chicken and vegetables moist.

Serve with unlimited vegetables of your choice or a salad.

Chicken Casserole

SERVES 1

1 x 175g (6oz) skinless chicken portion
(weighed with bone) or 1 x 115g (4oz) boned and
skinned chicken portion or breast
1 chicken stock cube
1 x 200g (7oz) can chopped tomatoes
150g (5oz) frozen casserole vegetables
½ teaspoon dried mixed herbs

Dissolve the stock cube in 50ml (2fl oz) boiling water.

Place the chicken portion or breast in a casserole dish. Add the stock, tomatoes, vegetables and herbs. Cover and bake in a preheated oven at 190C, 375F or Gas Mark 5 for 30–40 minutes until the chicken is tender. Alternatively, microwave on High for 10 minutes, stir, and cook for a further 10 minutes on Medium High.

Serve with 1 x 175g (6oz) jacket potato.

Chicken and Mushroom Pasta

SERVES 3

You could substitute 225g (8oz) diced turkey or pork for the chicken if you like.

1 medium onion, chopped
2 x 115g (2 x 4oz) boned and
skinned chicken breasts, cubed
115g (4oz) mushrooms, sliced
1 medium courgette, diced
1 small green pepper, diced
1 x 200g (7oz) can chopped tomatoes
1 x 295g (11oz) can Campbell's
Condensed Half Fat Mushroom Soup
$\frac{1}{4}$ teaspoon mixed herbs or to taste
salt and pepper
1 slice brown bread, made into crumbs
75g (3oz) [dry weight] pasta shapes of choice

Dry-fry the onion until nearly tender. Remove from the pan.

Dry-fry the chicken until golden brown. Return the onion to the pan and add the mushrooms, courgette and pepper and cook together for a few minutes.

Stir in the tomatoes, soup and herbs. Season to taste and leave to simmer gently until the vegetables are almost tender.

In the meantime, cook the pasta in boiling salted water. When cooked, drain well and add to the chicken mixture. Stir thoroughly and pour into an ovenproof dish. Sprinkle the breadcrumbs over and place in a preheated oven at 190C, 375F or Gas Mark

5 for 20 minutes or until the vegetables are tender. If you wish, you can pop the dish under a hot grill for a few minutes to brown.

Serve hot with a salad.

Chicken with Mushrooms

SERVES 2

2 x 115g (2 x 4oz) boned and
skinned chicken breasts
1 x 295g (11oz) can Campbell's
Condensed Half Fat Mushroom Soup
25g (1oz) mushrooms, sliced
25g (1oz) fresh breadcrumbs

To cook in a microwave, place the chicken breasts, mushroom soup and mushrooms in a microwave dish. Cover and cook in the microwave on High for 6 minutes. Turn the chicken breasts over and cook for a further 5 minutes. To test if the chicken is cooked, prick with a fork to make sure the juices from the chicken run clear.

Alternatively, to cook in a conventional oven, place the chicken and mushrooms in an ovenproof dish. Place the soup in a saucepan and bring to the boil. Pour the soup over the chicken and mushrooms. Cover and place in a preheated oven at 180C, 350F or Gas Mark 4 for 20–30 minutes or until the chicken is tender.

Once the chicken is cooked, sprinkle the breadcrumbs over the top and cook under a hot grill until golden brown. Serve with 175g (6oz) potatoes per person and a selection of mixed vegetables.

Chicken Paprika

SERVES 4

1 medium onion, chopped
4 x 115 g (4 x 4oz) boned and
skinned chicken breasts
salt and pepper
1 tablespoon flour
1 tablespoon paprika
1 tablespoon tomato purée
1 x 400g (14oz) can chopped tomatoes
1 x 150g (5oz) pot low-fat natural yogurt
115g (4oz) [dry weight] tagliatelle

Dry-fry the onion in a hot pan until it is translucent and lightly coloured. Remove from the pan and reserve.

Rub a little salt and pepper into the chicken and dry-fry the chicken until golden brown on both sides. Remove from the pan.

Return the onions to the pan. Add the flour, paprika and tomato purée. Stir well to mix. Add the tin of tomatoes, mix well and bring to the boil.

Return the chicken pieces to the pan and check the seasoning. Transfer the chicken and sauce to an ovenproof dish.

Cook in a preheated oven at 180C, 350F or Gas Mark 4 for 30–40 minutes or until the chicken and onions are tender.

When the chicken is cooked, stir in the yogurt and check the seasoning again. Allow to heat through without boiling.

In the meantime, cook the tagliatelle according to the instructions. Drain well.

Serve the chicken on a bed of tagliatelle with a green salad.

Chicken and Sweetcorn Roll

SERVES 4–5

450g (1lb) minced chicken
1 large onion, grated
1 large carrot, grated
75g (3oz) fresh white breadcrumbs
2 tablespoons Worcester sauce
2 tablespoons tomato purée
1 teaspoon mixed herbs
1 large egg
salt and pepper
1 x 326g (11½oz) can sweetcorn, drained

Mix all ingredients except the sweetcorn in a large bowl. Leave to stand for a few minutes.

Take a large piece of foil and cover with a piece of greaseproof or silicone paper. Place the chicken mixture in the centre of the paper and pat into a rectangle (25 x 20cm/10 x 8 inches). Spread the sweetcorn on top then, starting with one of the shorter sides and using the paper to help, roll up the mixture like a Swiss roll. Wrap the paper and then the foil around the roll and fold the ends over firmly to make a long parcel. Prick the bottom of the roll to allow any fat or liquid to drain away. Place on a baking tray and bake in a preheated oven at 200C, 400F or Gas Mark 6 for 1–1¼ hours.

When cooked, gently peel off the foil and paper and place the roll on a serving dish.

Serve with gravy made from low-fat chicken granules if desired, plus 175g (6oz) potatoes per person and mixed vegetables or a salad.

Chicken Tikka

SERVES 4

1 garlic clove, crushed
1 x 150g (5oz) pot low-fat natural yogurt
1 tablespoon tomato purée
1½ teaspoons cumin
1 teaspoon ground coriander
1 teaspoon turmeric
½–1 teaspoon chilli powder
½ teaspoon ground ginger
1 tablespoon chopped fresh coriander
salt
4 x 115g (4 x 4oz) boned and skinned chicken breasts

Make the marinade by mixing together all the ingredients except the chicken breasts and season to taste with salt.

Place the chicken in a shallow dish, coat with the marinade and leave for at least 2 hours.

Place the chicken on a wire rack in a roasting tin and bake in a preheated oven at 220C, 425F or Gas mark 7 for about 25 minutes or until cooked. Pierce with a skewer. If the juices run clear, the chicken is cooked.

Serve with boiled rice (allow 40g/1½oz dry weight per person) or 175g (6oz) jacket potatoes, plus salad.

Jambalaya

SERVES 4

Extra vegetables of your choice may be added to this dish, e.g. peas, courgettes, carrots. If you prefer to use fewer peppers, use half the quantity given.

2 x 115g (4oz) boned and skinned chicken breasts
175g (6oz) lean smoked bacon
1 bunch spring onions, chopped
1–2 garlic cloves, crushed
1 small red pepper, thinly sliced
1 small green pepper, thinly sliced
1 small yellow pepper, thinly sliced
115g (4oz) mushrooms, chopped
1 x 400g (14oz) can chopped tomatoes
1 x 115g (4oz) packet boil in the bag rice, cooked

Thinly slice the chicken. Remove any fat from the bacon and discard. Chop the bacon into pieces.

Dry-fry the onions and garlic in a hot heavy-based pan until soft. Remove from the pan.

Dry-fry the peppers, mushrooms and any other vegetables (if using). Remove from the pan.

Dry-fry the chicken and bacon until tender. Return the onions, garlic, peppers, mushrooms and other vegetables (if using) to the pan. Add the chopped tomatoes. Bring to the boil and, if necessary, cook for a few minutes until all the ingredients are tender but the vegetables should remain a little crunchy.

Add the cooked rice, heat through and serve.

Mediterranean Chicken

SERVES 4

115g (4oz) Thai Fragrant Rice
(or other long grain rice)
pinch of saffron
salt
4 bay leaves
4 x 115g (4oz) boned and skinned chicken breasts
250ml (8fl oz) white wine
3–4 shallots, finely chopped
2 garlic cloves, finely chopped
1 x 200g (7oz) can chopped tomatoes
1 tablespoon tomato purée
black pepper
1–2 tablespoons chopped fresh coriander

Wash the rice in 6 changes of cold water until the water is clear.

Bring a pan of water to the boil and add the rice, saffron, salt and 2 of the bay leaves. Bring to the boil, stir once, and boil uncovered for 12 minutes.

Drain, rinse the rice with cold water and drain again. Leave the rice to dry.

In the meantime, place the chicken breasts in a large frying pan. Pour the wine and an equal quantity of water into the pan. Add the shallots, the 2 remaining bay leaves and the garlic. Season with a little salt.

Cover the pan and poach the chicken breasts for about 20 minutes or until tender. Keep the heat low so that the chicken does not become tough and do not overcook.

In the meantime, reheat the rice. Place the rice in an ovenproof dish, cover tightly with foil and warm through in the oven at 180C, 350F or Gas Mark 4 for about 20 minutes. Alternatively, the rice can be reheated in the microwave for 3 minutes.

Remove the chicken from the pan, cover and keep warm in the oven. Discard the bay leaves and add the tomatoes, tomato purée, black pepper and 1 table-spoon of the chopped coriander. Bring to the boil and simmer until the sauce reduces. Check the seasoning.

Cut the chicken into thin strips, add to the sauce and cook for 1 minute.

Place the chicken on a bed of rice and, just before serving, sprinkle the remaining chopped coriander over. Serve with sweetcorn and mange-tout or other vegetables of your choice.

Pineapple and Cranberry Chicken

SERVES 4

4 x 115g (4oz) boned and skinned chicken breasts
1 x 425g (15oz) can pineapple slices
in pineapple juice
300ml (½ pint) cranberry juice
150ml (¼ pint) vegetable stock
salt and pepper
25g (1oz) cornflour

Place the chicken breasts in an ovenproof dish or casserole.

Drain the pineapple juice from the can into a saucepan. Add the cranberry juice and vegetable stock. Bring to the boil and season to taste with salt and pepper.

Place 2 pineapple slices on top of each chicken breast and then pour the juice and vegetable liquid over. Cover with foil or a tight-fitting lid and bake in a pre-heated oven at 190C, 375F or Gas Mark 5 for 1 hour.

Remove the foil or the lid and drain the liquid into a pan. Cover the chicken again and return it to the oven.

Slake the cornflour with a little cold water and pour into the liquid. Bring to the boil, stirring continuously, and boil for 2–3 minutes. Check the seasoning then pour the sauce over the chicken.

Return the chicken to the oven for another 10 minutes.

Serve with minted peas, Pinto Bean Salad (page 170) and 175g (6oz) Dry-roast Potatoes (page 167) per person.

Sticky Ginger Chicken

SERVES 4

2 tablespoons lemon juice
2 tablespoons light muscavado sugar
1 teaspoon grated fresh ginger root
2 teaspoons soy sauce
freshly ground pepper
salt to taste (optional)
8 chicken drumsticks or thighs

Mix together the lemon juice, sugar, ginger, soy sauce and pepper to form a glaze. Taste and add a little salt if you wish.

Remove the skin and any fat from the drumsticks or thighs. Slash the flesh on each one 2–3 times and toss in the glaze.

Cook under a moderately hot grill or on a barbecue until the chicken juices are clear when the flesh is pierced with a skewer. Turn the chicken pieces occasionally and brush them with the glaze.

Serve with a crispy salad or unlimited vegetables.

Surprise, Surprise Chicken

SERVES 3

It is not essential to marinate the chicken in this recipe, but it does add flavour. You can also use slices of turkey breast instead of chicken.

3 x 115–175g (3 x 4–6oz) boned and
skinned chicken breasts or portions
1 x 150g (5oz) pot low-fat natural yogurt
2 teaspoons Tandoori spice
1 teaspoon lemon juice
1 can Diet Coke
1 packet mushroom or potato and leek soup mix
225g (8oz) mushrooms, halved
1 teaspoon cornflour or
low-fat gravy granules (optional)

Cut the chicken breasts or portions into 3–4 pieces, slantwise.

Mix the yogurt with the Tandoori spice and lemon juice. Pour over the chicken pieces and mix well. Cover with cling film and leave in the refrigerator for at least 2 hours or overnight.

Drain the marinade from the chicken. Place the chicken in an ovenproof casserole and sprinkle the dry soup mix over. Add the Diet Coke (it will fizz) and stir to mix.

Place in a preheated oven at 200C, 400F or Gas Mark 6 and cook for 45–60 minutes or until the chicken is tender. Stir occasionally.

Ten minutes before the end of cooking time, add the mushrooms and mix in well.

When the chicken and mushrooms are tender, remove from the oven and thicken the sauce with cornflour or low-fat gravy granules.

Serve with boiled rice (allow 25g/1oz dry weight per person) and unlimited fresh vegetables.

Seasoned Chicken Portions

SERVES 2

2 x 115g (2 x 4oz) boned and
skinned chicken portions
salt and freshly ground black pepper
¼ teaspoon dried mixed herbs
½ medium onion, thinly sliced
50g (2oz) mushrooms, sliced

Cut 2 large pieces of foil and place them shiny side up. Place a chicken portion on each and season with salt and pepper.

Divide the herbs, onions and mushrooms between the 2 pieces.

Wrap the foil around the chicken, making sure that all the edges are sealed.

Place on a baking sheet and bake in a preheated oven at 190C, 375F or Gas Mark 5 for 45 minutes.

Serve with 175g (6oz) new potatoes per person and unlimited vegetables of your choice.

Stuffed Chicken Breasts

SERVES 4

4 x 115g (4 x 4oz) boned and
skinned chicken breasts
¼ small red pepper
¼ small green pepper
¼ large carrot
1 medium onion
6 medium white mushrooms
1–2 tablespoons low-fat fromage frais
1 tablespoon chopped fresh coriander or tarragon
salt and pepper
2–3 teaspoons lemon juice
300ml (½ pint) chicken stock
300ml (½ pint) skimmed milk
15g (½oz) cornflour

Remove the fillet from the back of each chicken breast and, using a sharp knife, scrape out the thick white sinew and discard. Reserve the fillets.

Place the chicken breasts on a board and, using a knife, cut through each breast from the thick side until you can open it out like an escalope.

Place a fillet in the centre of each breast, cover with a piece of cling film or greaseproof paper and hammer the breast out gently with a rolling pin.

Chop the vegetables finely and place half in a bowl. Add sufficient fromage frais to bind and half the chopped coriander or tarragon. Season with salt and pepper. Place a portion on each chicken breast, roll up and secure each one with a small skewer or cock-tail stick.

Place each chicken roll on a square of aluminium foil. Season lightly and sprinkle the lemon juice over the top. Roll up each piece of chicken in the foil and seal tightly. Place in a baking tin and cook in a pre-heated oven at 180C, 350F or Gas Mark 4 for 35–45 minutes or until tender.

In the meantime, cook the remainder of the veget-ables, except for the mushrooms, in the stock. When most of the liquid has evaporated, add the mush-rooms and cook for a further 2–3 minutes.

When the chicken is cooked, make a white sauce. Pour a little of the milk onto the cornflour and mix well. Heat the remainder of the milk in the saucepan until hot but not boiling. Slowly pour some of the hot milk onto the cornflour mixture, stirring continu-ously. Gradually stir in the rest of the milk. Mix the sauce well again and return to the pan with any resid-ual stock from the vegetables. Bring to the boil, stir-ring continuously, and cook for 2–3 minutes, still stirring. Add the vegetables and the remainder of the chopped herbs and season to taste with salt and pepper.

Remove the chicken breasts from the foil and remove the skewers or cocktail sticks. Arrange on a hot serving dish, pour a little sauce over and serve the rest separately.

Serve with 175g (6oz) potatoes per person and unlimited vegetables.

Tasty Citrus Chicken Parcels

SERVES 6

6 x 115g (6 x 4oz) boned and
skinned chicken breasts
4 garlic cloves, chopped
1½ teaspoons salt
1 teaspoon chopped oregano
1 teaspoon ground cumin
1 teaspoon freshly ground black pepper
4 tablespoons orange juice
4 tablespoons lemon juice
4 tablespoons lime juice

Dry the chicken pieces with a paper towel and place in a large bowl.

Combine the garlic, salt, oregano, cumin, pepper and fruit juices. Pour over the chicken, cover and place in the refrigerator. Leave to marinate for 24 hours, turning 2 or 3 times.

Cut 6 pieces of aluminium foil (approx. 30cm/12 inches square). Place a chicken breast on each square. Spoon the marinade equally over each one, holding up the edges of the foil to avoid any spillage. Fold the foil over the chicken and seal the edges tightly.

Arrange the foil dishes in a baking dish and bake in a preheated oven at 180C, 350F or Gas Mark 4 for 1½ hours or until the chicken is tender and the juices run clear. After an hour, open one of the parcels carefully and check.

When cooked, slit open the parcels. Serve with 175g (6oz) jacket potatoes per person and unlimited vegetables.

Spicy Chicken or Turkey Burgers

SERVES 4

450g (1lb) minced chicken or turkey
115g (4oz) firm mushrooms, grated
1 medium carrot, grated
1 medium leek, quartered and finely sliced
1 egg
1 egg white
½ teaspoon dried ginger
1 teaspoon curry powder
pinch of cayenne pepper or to taste
salt
finely chopped fresh basil to taste

Mix all the ingredients together well to bind. Turn out onto a floured board. Divide the mixture into 8 and mould into burger shapes.

Cook under medium hot grill for 8–10 minutes each side until golden brown on both sides.

Serve with a crisp salad, plus 175g (6oz) jacket potatoes or a wholemeal bap per person and tomato sauce.

Apricot Turkey Beanfeast

SERVES 4

4 new potatoes
salt
2 sticks celery, diced
1 medium onion, diced
4 x 115g (4 x 4oz) turkey breast steaks
2 tablespoons apricot jam
300ml (½ pint) chicken stock
2 teaspoons tomato purée
1 teaspoon garlic purée
1 x 400g (14oz) can mixed beans, drained
1 heaped teaspoon arrowroot
115g (4oz) [dry weight] rice
1 pilau rice stock cube

Peel the potatoes and boil in salted water until nearly tender. Drain well and cut into quarters.

In the meantime, heat a non-stick or heavy-based pan. Add the celery and onion and dry-fry gently until the onion starts to colour. Remove from the pan and reserve.

Place the turkey steaks in the pan and cook until coloured on both sides. Remove from the pan and return the celery and onion to the pan. Add the apricot jam. Remove the pan from the heat, cover and leave for 5 minutes until the jam has melted.

Mix the stock, tomato purée and garlic purée into the pan.

Stir well and season lightly.

Return the turkey steaks to the pan, cover and simmer for about 5 minutes.

Add the potatoes and continue cooking for a further 15 minutes. Five minutes before the end of the cooking time, add the mixed beans. Mix the arrowroot with a little water, add to the sauce in the pan and bring to the boil stirring continuously. Check the seasoning.

In the meantime, cook the rice according to the instructions, using the pilau rice stock cube.

When the rice is cooked, pile it onto a serving plate and make a big well in the centre. Arrange the turkey steaks in the centre of the dish and pour the sauce over.

If desired, serve with a little natural yogurt.

Exotic Turkey

SERVES 4–6

This is a rather hot curry. If you prefer a milder one, reduce the amount of chillies or chilli powder and Madras curry powder.

2 large onions, finely chopped
4 chillies, finely chopped, or
1 teaspoon chilli powder
3 tablespoons Madras curry powder
6 tablespoons white wine vinegar
6 tablespoons tomato purée
1 teaspoon turmeric
½ teaspoon mustard powder
1½ teaspoons sugar
450–675g (1–1½lb) raw diced turkey

Place all the ingredients in a bowl and mix well. Leave to marinate for about 2 hours.

Add a cup of water and mix well again. Place the mixture in a saucepan, bring to the boil and simmer gently for about 1 hour or until the meat is tender. Add a little more water if the mixture becomes too dry.

Serve hot with boiled rice (allow 25g/1oz dry weight per person) mixed with canned or fresh beansprouts, plus unlimited vegetables.

Grilled Breast of Turkey in a Basil and Mushroom Sauce

SERVES 2

225g (8oz) turkey breast fillet
1 chicken stock cube
1 teaspoon Dijon mustard (optional)
1 small onion, chopped
1 teaspoon dried basil or
2 teaspoons chopped fresh basil
175g (6oz) button mushrooms
2 teaspoons cornflour
1 tablespoon Worcester sauce

Cut the turkey into 4 equal portions.

Preheat a heavy-cast grillade or heavy based pan and cook the turkey for 3–4 minutes on each side until brown. Remove from the pan.

Dissolve the chicken stock cube in 300ml (½ pint) boiling water. Pour the stock into the pan or, if you are using a grillade, into a clean pan.

Rub the Dijon mustard (if using) into the turkey pieces. Return the turkey to the pan. Add the onion and basil and cook gently for 15–20 minutes, adding the mushrooms for the last 5–7 minutes.

Mix the cornflour with a little cold water and stir into the sauce. Add the Worcester sauce. Bring to the boil and simmer for a further 2–3 minutes, stirring continuously to prevent the sauce from becoming lumpy.

Serve hot with 175g (6oz) new potatoes per person and a selection of vegetables such as a julienne of carrots, sliced courgettes and broccoli spears. If you wish, you can pour the sauce over the vegetables and sprinkle some fresh mint or parsley over the potatoes.

Turkey Bake

SERVES 4

450g (1lb) minced turkey
1 onion, finely chopped
1–2 garlic cloves, crushed
1 teaspoon cinnamon powder
1 teaspoon cumin powder
1 red pepper, chopped
1 x 400g (14oz) can chopped tomatoes
150ml (¼ pint) white wine or chicken stock
salt and pepper
25g (1oz) plain flour
300ml (½ pint) skimmed milk from allowance
½ stock cube
1 x 200g (7oz) can sweetcorn, drained
25g (1oz) fresh breadcrumbs
½ teaspoon paprika

Dry-fry the turkey mince, onion and garlic until browned.

Add the cinnamon, cumin, chopped pepper, tomatoes and wine or stock. Season to taste, bring to the boil and simmer for 20 minutes.

Mix the flour with a little of the milk to form a paste. Gradually add more milk, whisking all the time with a balloon whisk, until all the milk has been added. Add the stock cube and bring to the boil over a moderate heat, still whisking, and cook for 2–3 minutes until thick and creamy. Check the seasoning.

Place the turkey mixture in an ovenproof dish, cover with the sweetcorn and pour over the sauce.

Mix the breadcrumbs and paprika together and sprinkle them over the top.

Bake in a preheated oven at 200C, 400F or Gas Mark 6 for 30 minutes until golden brown.

Serve with a green salad or unlimited vegetables of your choice.

Turkey Bolognese

SERVES 2

175g (6oz) turkey mince
1 chicken stock cube
1 x 200g (7oz) can chopped tomatoes
½ jar bolognese sauce
50g (2oz) baked beans
1 teaspoon tomato purée
½ garlic clove, crushed, or
1 teaspoon garlic purée (optional)

Place the turkey mince in a hot heavy-based pan and dry-fry until the meat is golden brown.

Sprinkle the stock cube over and add the remaining ingredients. Bring to the boil and simmer for 30 minutes.

Serve with pasta (allow 50g/2oz dry weight per person) or 175g (6oz) jacket potatoes per person, plus unlimited vegetables or salad.

Fish Main Courses

Cod in Mustard Sauce

SERVES 2

2 x 150–250g (2 x 6–8oz) pieces cod
salt and white pepper
300ml (½ pint) skimmed milk (from allowance)
approx. 2 teaspoons cornflour
2 tablespoons skimmed milk powder
1 teaspoon English mustard or to taste
50g (2oz) fresh breadcrumbs

Place the cod in an ovenproof dish and season with salt and white pepper.

Heat most of the milk and pour over the cod. Cover and place in a preheated oven at 180C, 350F or Gas Mark 4 for 15–20 minutes or until cooked.

Mix the remaining milk with the cornflour and skimmed milk powder.

When the fish is cooked, remove it carefully from the dish.

Pour off the milk into a saucepan and return the fish to the cooking dish or a serving dish. Cover and keep hot.

Bring the milk in the saucepan to the boil, then pour it onto the cornflour mixture. Return the milk to the saucepan and bring to the boil, continuously. Boil for 2–3 minutes. Season to taste with salt, pepper and the mustard. Pour over the fish and sprinkle the breadcrumbs on top. Place under a hot grill to brown.

Serve with 175g (6oz) potatoes per person and unlimited vegetables of your choice.

If you prefer to cook the fish in the microwave, place the cod into a microwave dish, cover and microwave for 4–5 minutes on High or until cooked. Make the sauce and finish the dish as above.

Cod with Wine

SERVES 4

1 medium onion, thinly sliced
1 small garlic clove, crushed
1 x 400g (14oz) can chopped tomatoes
1 tablespoon chopped parsley
1 level tablespoon plain flour
2 rounded teaspoons non-fat milk powder
2 tablespoons white wine or
2 teaspoons Worcester sauce
1 tablespoon lemon juice
salt and pepper
4 x 175–200g (4 x 6–7oz) cod steaks

Place the onion, garlic, tomatoes and parsley in a saucepan and simmer until the onion is soft.

Mix the flour and milk powder together with a little water to make a thin paste. Stir this into the mixture in the saucepan.

Add the wine or the Worcester sauce and the lemon juice and season lightly with salt and pepper. Bring to the boil and pour into an ovenproof dish.

Season the cod steaks and place them on top of the tomato mixture. Cover and bake in a preheated oven at 190C, 375F or Gas Mark 5 for 20–25 minutes.

When cooked, check the seasoning and serve with 175g (6oz) potatoes per person and vegetables of your choice.

Pasta Twirls with Scallops and Bacon

SERVES 4

4 lean rashers smoked back bacon
1 garlic clove, crushed
2 leeks, thinly sliced
1 x 200g (7oz) can tomatoes
150ml (¼ pint) white wine
6 large mushrooms, diced
salt and pepper
175g (6oz) scallops
115g (4oz) [dry weight] pasta twirls

Trim all the fat from the bacon and discard. Cut the bacon into strips. Dry-fry the bacon in a non-stick pan until almost tender but without colour. Drain off any fat.

Add the garlic and cook for a moment or two.

Add the tomatoes, white wine and mushrooms. Season to taste. Bring to the boil and simmer for about 8 minutes.

Add the scallops and continue cooking for a further 1–2 minutes until the mushrooms are tender and the sauce has reduced. Scallops need only a little cooking, just until they become opaque (they are better undercooked than overcooked or they will become tough).

In the meantime, cook the pasta according to the instructions. Drain well and stir into the sauce.

Pile into a hot serving dish and serve.

Poached Salmon with Dill Sauce

SERVES 4

4 x 150g (4 x 5oz) salmon steaks or fillets
4 spring onions, chopped
2 tablespoons white wine
juice of ½ lemon
2 thick slices lemon
salt and pepper

for the sauce
1 heaped tablespoon cornflour
liquid from poached salmon made up to 300ml
(½ pint) with fish stock or
skimmed milk from allowance
2 tablespoons chopped fresh dill
3 tablespoons low-fat fromage frais
salt and pepper

Place the salmon in a microwave dish. Sprinkle the spring onions, wine and lemon juice over the salmon. Add the lemon slices. Season lightly with salt and pepper. Cover with cling film and pierce holes in the film. Cook on high for 4 minutes or until cooked. Leave to cool or keep warm depending on your choice.

If you prefer to cook the salmon in a conventional oven, place the fish in an ovenproof dish, add all the flavourings, cover with a tight-fitting lid or foil and bake in a preheated oven at 180C, 350F or Gas Mark 4 for 12–15 minutes or until tender.

To make the sauce, mix the cornflour with a little water in a small pan. Add the fish stock and/or milk. Bring to the boil, stirring continuously.

Add the chopped dill and simmer for 3–4 minutes, stirring steadily. Just before serving, stir in the fromage frais. Taste and add more seasoning if necessary.

Serve with hot or cold salmon and new or Dry-roast Potatoes (page 167), seasonal vegetables or green salad.

Quick and Easy Salmon with Dill

SERVES 4

4 x 150g (4 x 5oz) salmon steaks
juice from ½ lemon
salt and pepper
2 tablespoons low-fat fromage frais
½ teaspoon mustard powder
1 tablespoon finely chopped fresh dill

Sprinkle the salmon with the lemon juice and season lightly with salt and pepper. Grill for 5–8 minutes on each side until brown or microwave on High for 8–9 minutes.

Mix the fromage frais with the mustard powder and dill and serve with the salmon.

Serve with 175g (6oz) new potatoes per person and a mixed salad or unlimited vegetables of your choice.

Salmon Olives in Asparagus Sauce

SERVES 2

2 x 150–225g (5–8oz) tail fillets of salmon, skinned
coarse grained mustard to taste
2–3 tablespoons lemon juice or to taste
freshly ground black pepper
1 x 295g (11oz) can Campbell's Condensed
Half Fat Asparagus Soup
1 x 411g (14oz) can asparagus tips, coarsely chopped
150ml (¼ pint) dry white wine
chopped fresh dill to taste

Place the salmon fillets on a board. Press down lightly with one hand and, using a sharp knife, slice through each fillet from the tail end to make two slices. Spread the skin side of each slice with the mustard, roll up and secure carefully with cocktail sticks.

Place the salmon olives in an ovenproof dish, sprinkle the lemon juice over and season well with black pepper. Cover with a tight-fitting lid or foil and cook in a preheated oven at 180C, 375F or Gas Mark 5 for 15–20 minutes or until the fish is tender.

Heat the soup and asparagus tips with the white wine in a saucepan. Add the chopped dill (reserve some for the garnish) and simmer gently for about 10 minutes. If the sauce is too thick, add some more wine or a little water.

Pour a little sauce onto 2 plates. Remove the cocktail sticks from the salmon olives and place the olives on top of the sauce.

Sprinkle a little more fresh dill over the top and serve with 175g (6oz) potatoes per person and fresh vegetables. Serve any extra sauce separately.

Special Fish Stir-fry

SERVES 2

1 x 450g (1lb) rainbow trout
1 tablespoon soy sauce
2 tablespoons sherry or rice wine
1 large field mushroom, diced
$\frac{1}{2}$ red pepper, diced
$\frac{1}{2}$ green pepper, diced
$\frac{1}{2}$ large onion, diced
4 baby sweetcorn, sliced
2 small carrots, sliced
6 mange-tout, halved
1 garlic clove, crushed (optional)
salt and pepper

Remove the head, skin and bones from the fish and discard. Flake or cut the fish into small pieces.

Heat a wok or heavy-based pan, pour in the soy sauce and sherry or rice wine and add all the vegetables and the garlic (if using). Mix well and season to taste with salt and pepper. Cover with a tight-fitting lid and cook for 5 minutes.

Uncover the pan, add the fish and cook for a further 5 minutes until the fish is cooked.

Check the seasoning and add a little more soy sauce if desired.

Serve with cooked rice noodles (allow 75–115g/3–4oz total weight) or 115g (4oz) new potatoes, plus unlimited vegetables.

Tuna Pasta

SERVES 2

2 x 400g (2 x 14oz) cans tomatoes
1 small onion, chopped very fine
115g (4oz) mushrooms, sliced
dried mixed herbs to taste
salt and black pepper
115g (4oz) [dry weight] pasta shapes
1 x 200g (7oz) can tuna chunks in spring water, drained and flaked

Place the tomatoes (including their juice) into a saucepan. Add the onion, mushrooms and dried herbs. Season lightly. Bring to the boil, then reduce the heat and simmer until the onion is tender and the sauce has thickened slightly. When the sauce is nearly ready, cook the pasta according to the instructions.

Add the flaked tuna to the sauce and warm through. Drain the pasta shapes well and add to the sauce. Mix well together and check the seasoning. Serve hot with a side salad.

Tuna Risotto

SERVES 4

250g (9oz) [dry weight] brown rice
1 garlic clove, crushed
½–1 teaspoon chilli powder
6 cardamom pods
2–3 teaspoons garam masala
2 x 200g (2 x 7oz) cans tuna steak in water
1 medium onion, chopped
1 x 400g (14oz) can chopped tomatoes
200g (7oz) mushrooms, cut into large pieces
2 tablespoons tomato purée
2 medium carrots, cut into fine matchsticks
salt

Wash the rice and cook in boiling salted water for 20–30 minutes until almost tender. Drain well.

In the meantime, place the garlic, chilli powder, cardamom pods and garam masala in a hot heavy-based pan and heat through for a moment or two.

Drain the water from the tuna into the pan and boil for about a minute. Add the chopped onion, tomatoes, mushrooms and tomato purée. Season to taste. Bring to the boil and simmer until the onions are tender.

Add the tuna, carrots and cooked rice. Cook for another 7–10 minutes until the rice is tender, the carrots are slightly crunchy and the sauce has reduced enough to coat the rice without being runny. Stir frequently at this stage to prevent the rice from sticking to the bottom of the pan.

Serve with a green salad.

Variation If you wish you can substitute your favourite seasoning or mixed herbs for the chilli powder, cardamom pods and garam masala, and use other vegetables (e.g. courgettes, peppers, peas) as well as or in place of the carrots.

Tuna Chilli Tacos

SERVES 4

8 taco shells
1 x 425g (15oz) can red kidney beans
120ml (4fl oz) low-fat fromage frais
½ teaspoon chilli sauce
2 spring onions, chopped
1 teaspoon chopped fresh mint
½ small crisp lettuce, shredded
1 x 425g (15oz) can tuna in brine, drained
8 cherry tomatoes, quartered

Warm the taco shells in a hot oven for a few minutes until crisp.

Drain and rinse the red kidney beans then mash them with a fork. Stir in the fromage frais, chilli sauce, spring onions and mint.

Fill the shells with the shredded lettuce, bean mix and tuna. Serve immediately with the quartered tomatoes and unlimited salad.

Tuna Quiche

SERVES 4

2 x 185g (2 x 6½oz) can tuna in brine, drained
1 medium onion, chopped
115g (4oz) sweetcorn
115g (4oz) mushrooms
115g (4oz) cooked peas
1 small red pepper, chopped
1 x 227g (8oz) tub low-fat cottage cheese
1 egg
1 tablespoon skimmed milk
salt and pepper
2–3 tomatoes to garnish

Use the tuna to line a pie dish. Press the tuna firmly round the base and up the sides. Arrange the vegetables on top of the tuna.

Sieve the cottage cheese, or purée in a food processor or liquidiser and beat in the egg and milk. Season to taste and pour over the tuna and vegetables.

Slice the tomatoes and arrange over the top of the sauce. Bake in a preheated oven at 180C, 350F or Gas Mark 4 for approximately 40 minutes until the cheese is set.

Serve hot or cold with jacket potatoes (115g/4oz per person) and salad.

Tuna Curry

SERVES 4

1 large onion, finely chopped
3 garlic cloves, crushed
1 teaspoon grated fresh ginger root
$\frac{1}{2}$–1 teaspoon finely chopped green chilli or to taste
$\frac{1}{2}$ teaspoon turmeric
1 x 200g (7oz) can chopped tomatoes
$\frac{1}{2}$ teaspoon salt
1 teaspoon garam masala
$\frac{1}{2}$ teaspoon tomato purée
300g (11oz) canned tuna in brine, drained
2 tablespoons sweetcorn
1 tablespoon chopped fresh coriander

Dry-fry the onion until slightly golden brown. Add the garlic, ginger and chilli and cook for a few minutes, stirring all the time. Add the turmeric and stir in well. Add the chopped tomatoes and tomato purée and simmer over a low heat for approximately 10 minutes, stirring occasionally. Add the salt and garam masala and continue cooking over a low heat for 5–7 minutes. Finally flake the tuna. Add the tuna and the sweetcorn to the mixture and cook for a further 5–7 minutes.

Just before serving, stir in the chopped coriander.

Serve with boiled brown rice (allow 25g/1oz dry weight per person) mixed with canned or fresh beansprouts, plus 2 tablespoons low-fat natural yogurt per person and unlimited vegetables of your choice.

Haddock and Tomato Hotpot

SERVES 4

1 large onion, sliced
1 garlic clove, crushed
2 x 400g (14oz) cans chopped tomatoes
3 tablespoons tomato purée
1 large courgette, sliced
2 teaspoons sugar
2 tablespoons lemon juice
salt and freshly ground black pepper
675g (1½lb) haddock fillets, skinned and flaked
115g (4oz) button mushrooms
450g (1lb) potatoes, sliced 5mm (¼ inch) thick
and cooked

Gently sauté the onion in a non-stick frying pan until the onion is soft and transparent. Add the crushed garlic, tomatoes, tomato puree, courgette, sugar and lemon juice and simmer for 15 minutes. Season the tomato mixture and stir in the fish and mushrooms.

Transfer the mixture to an ovenproof dish and arrange the potato slices over the top. Cook in a preheated oven at 200C, 400F or Gas Mark 6 for 30 minutes or until the potatoes are golden brown.

Serve with unlimited green vegetables.

Vegetarian Main Courses

Cheesy Bean and Swede Layer

SERVES 1

25g (1oz) canned red kidney beans
25g (1oz) canned black-eyed beans
25g (1oz) canned mung beans
50ml (2fl oz) tomato juice
a little chopped fresh parsley
salt and pepper
115g (4oz) cooked and mashed swede (kept hot)
25g (1oz) grated low-fat cheese

Place the beans in a microwave dish or a saucepan. Mix the tomato juice, parsley and seasoning together and pour over the beans. Cover and cook in the microwave on High for 2–3 minutes, or heat through on top of the stove.

If cooking in a pan, transfer the mixture to a heat-proof dish. Spread the cooked swede over the beans, sprinkle with the cheese and place under the grill to brown.

Chinese Vegetable Stir-fry

SERVES 4

175g (6oz) American easy-cook rice
2 large carrots, cut into small matchsticks
1 large onion, sliced
1 x 325g (11½oz) can sweetcorn
3 celery sticks, cut into small matchsticks
1 large red pepper, cut into small matchsticks
1 large green pepper, cut into small matchsticks
225g (8oz) button mushrooms, sliced
2 Oxo Chinese stir-fry cubes
½ small Chinese leaf lettuce, shredded
soy sauce
1 x 400g (14oz) can beansprouts

Cook the rice according to the instructions. Drain well.

Place the carrots and onion in a large pan and add a little water or the juice from the sweetcorn. Place a lid on the pan and cook quickly, stirring frequently.

When the carrots and onions are almost cooked, add the celery, peppers, mushrooms and crumbled Oxo cubes. Finally, add the lettuce and sweetcorn. If the stir-fry becomes too dry, add some soy sauce or a little water.

Drain the beansprouts. Heat through in a saucepan or a microwave. When hot, mix with the cooked rice.

Serve the stir-fry on a bed of the rice and beansprouts with soy sauce, if desired.

Continental Lentil Curry

SERVES 3

225g (8oz) Continental (green) lentils
1 large onion, chopped
2 garlic cloves, crushed
2 teaspoons ginger
2 teaspoons ground coriander
2 teaspoons ground cumin
salt and pepper

Soak the lentils for several hours or overnight in cold water.

Rinse well then place in a pan and cover with water. Simmer for about 40 minutes or until tender. Drain.

Dry-fry the onion and garlic for 5 minutes. Add the ginger, coriander and cumin and cook for a further 5 minutes, adding a little water if necessary. Season to taste with salt and pepper.

Combine the lentil mixture with the onion mixture and heat through.

Serve with boiled rice (allow 50g/2oz dry weight per person) and mango chutney or with low-fat Naan bread and a tomato salad.

Variation Other vegetables can be added to the curry for colour and texture (e.g. chopped peppers, mushrooms, celery, sweetcorn). Add to the pan with the onion and garlic and a little water and cook gently.

Vegetarians and maintenance dieters may also add a few peanuts to the curry.

Couscous Salad

SERVES 4

250g (9oz) easy-to-cook couscous
1 apple
50g (2oz) peanuts (vegetarians only)
25g (1oz) sultanas and raisins
1 red pepper, chopped
1 green pepper, chopped
1 medium onion, chopped
2 sticks celery, chopped
1 x 325g (11½oz) can sweetcorn, drained
1 x 400g (14oz) can kidney beans or chick peas
salt and pepper
soy sauce (optional)

Place the couscous into a large bowl, cover with boiling water and leave to soak for about 10 minutes.

Peel, core and chop the apple. Add to the couscous. Mix in the peanuts (if using), the dried fruit, peppers, onion, celery, sweetcorn and the kidney beans or chick peas. Season with salt and pepper.

Chill for half an hour.

If desired, pour a little soy sauce over the couscous before serving. Serve with crusty bread (50g/2oz per person), green salad 75g (3oz) low-fat cottage cheese per person.

Garlicky Stuffing and Lentil Layer

SERVES 4

175g (6oz) red lentils
175g (6oz) [dry weight] pasta bows
1 large onion, chopped
2 garlic cloves, crushed
1 large carrot, diced
2 sticks celery, chopped
2 green or red peppers, chopped
1 x 200g (7oz) can plum tomatoes
2 tablespoons tomato purée
1 vegetable stock cube
salt and pepper
1 x 85g (3¼oz) packet garlic and herb stuffing mix

Rinse the lentils. Place in a pan and cover with water. Cook for about 20 minutes until tender. Drain.

Meanwhile, cook the pasta according to the instructions. Drain well.

Place the onion, garlic and carrot in a pan with a little water, cover and simmer until the carrot is almost cooked. Add the celery and peppers to the pan and cook for a couple of minutes.

Combine the vegetables with the lentils, tomatoes, tomato purée, stock cube and seasoning in a large pan and heat through gently.

Make up the stuffing mix, adding half as much water again as indicated on the packet, as the stuffing needs to be fairly sloppy.

Place a layer of cooked pasta in the base of a large ovenproof dish. Follow with a layer of lentil mixture then a thin layer of stuffing. Continue like this and finish with a layer of stuffing.

Fork the top and bake in a preheated oven at 200C, 400F or Gas Mark 6 for 20 minutes until brown and crisp. Serve with broccoli and cauliflower florets.

Lentil and Potato Pie

SERVES 3

175g (6oz) red lentils
1 large onion, chopped
350g (12oz) potatoes
2 tablespoons pickle
1 teaspoon mixed herbs
salt and pepper
paprika

Rinse the lentils. Place the lentils and onion in a pan, cover with water and cook slowly for about 20 minutes until the lentils are tender and all water is absorbed.

Cook the potatoes in boiling salted water. Drain well and mash. Beat the mashed potato into the lentils. Add the pickle, herbs and plenty of salt and pepper and mix well.

Place the mixture in a shallow ovenproof dish. Fork the top and sprinkle a little paprika over the top. Bake in a preheated oven at 200C, 400F or Gas Mark 6 for 20 minutes until crisp and brown.

Serve with green vegetables and tomato sauce or with a green salad, plus crusty bread (allow 50g/2oz bread per person).

Pitta Cassoulet

SERVES 4–6

1 x 425g (15oz) can flageolet beans
1 x 425g (15oz) can black-eyed beans
1 x 425g (15oz) can pinto or red kidney beans
500ml (18fl oz) tomato Passata
2 garlic cloves, crushed
2 teaspoons dried tarragon
1 large onion, chopped
3 celery sticks, chopped
salt and pepper
175g (6oz) bulgar wheat
6 wholemeal pitta breads

Rinse all the beans under cold water.

Mix all the ingredients except the pitta bread and bulgar wheat together in a large pan. Simmer slowly for 30 minutes, stirring occasionally.

Add the bulgar wheat and cook for a further 10–15 minutes, stirring frequently.

Warm the pitta breads in the oven and slit each one open.

Use a slotted spoon to fill each pitta bread with the bean mixture.

Serve with a green salad.

Quick Pasta in Creamy Tomato, Onion and Mushroom Sauce

SERVES 2-3

1 x 400g (14oz) can chopped tomatoes
1 medium onion, chopped
pinch of salt
ground black pepper
good pinch of herbes de Provence
175g (6oz) [dry weight] pasta
115g (4oz) button mushrooms, sliced
50g (2oz) quark

Place the tomatoes in a wok. Add the onion, salt, pepper and herbs. Bring to the boil and simmer for 10 minutes.

Cook the pasta for approximately 12 minutes until slightly al dente.

Add the mushrooms to the tomato mixture and simmer for a further 2 minutes.

Stir in the quark to thicken the sauce.

Drain the pasta and stir into the sauce.

Serve with green salad or vegetables of your choice.

Quorn Pieces in French White Wine and Dill Sauce

SERVES 1

1 small onion, sliced
175g (6oz) Quorn pieces
½ tablespoon vegetable oil
1 x 300g (11oz) can Weight Watchers from Heinz
French White Wine and Dill Cooking Sauce
75g (3oz) [dry weight] rice

Cook the onions and Quorn pieces in the vegetable oil until brown. Stir in the cooking sauce and heat gently for about 15–20 minutes.

While the Quorn mixture is cooking, cook the rice according to the instructions. Drain well.

Pour the Quorn mixture over the cooked rice and serve immediately.

Stir-fry Quorn

SERVES 1

½ teaspoon sunflower oil
115g (4oz) Quorn chunks
2–3 spring onions, chopped
50g (2oz) red or green pepper, chopped
50g (2oz) baby corn
50g (2oz) mange-tout
1 medium carrot, cut in julienne strips
grated root ginger grated
65–100ml (2½–5fl oz) vegetable stock
1–2 teaspoons soy sauce
freshly ground black pepper

Heat the oil in a wok or non-stick pan. Add the Quorn and spring onions and cook for a few minutes.

Add the chopped pepper, the remaining vegetables and the grated ginger. Pour in a little of the stock and add the soy sauce. Continue to cook until the Quorn and vegetables are cooked but the vegetables are still crunchy. Add more stock as necessary to prevent the vegetables from sticking, but do not add too much at a time or the vegetables will become soggy (you may not need to use all the stock).

Season to taste and serve immediately.

Vegetable Goulash

SERVES 4

1 medium onion
75g (3oz) soya chunks
1 large onion, chopped
75g (3oz) carrots, sliced
1 red pepper, chopped
75g (3oz) potatoes, cut into chunks
1 x 400g (14oz) can tomatoes
300ml (½ pint) vegetable stock
2 bay leaves
2 teaspoons paprika
3 tablespoons low-fat natural yogurt
salt and freshly ground black pepper

Soak the soya chunks in 2 cupfuls of boiling water for 10 minutes, then drain well.

Place all the ingredients except the yogurt in a saucepan. Add 300ml (½ pint) water and bring to the boil. Cover and simmer for about an hour. Stir in the yogurt, and season to taste.

Serve with boiled brown rice (50g/2oz dry weight per person).

Vegetable Winter Bake

SERVES 4–5

225g (8oz) carrots, diced
225g (8oz) swede, diced
450–675g (1–1½lb) potatoes, quartered
(red potatoes are best)
salt and pepper
1–2 leeks, sliced
1 x 325g (11½oz) can sweetcorn, drained
3 large fresh tomatoes, quartered
1 teaspoon mixed herbs
a few cardamom pods, crushed
3 tablespoons sage and onion stuffing mix
50g (2oz) grated low-fat Cheddar cheese

for the sauce
50g (2oz) plain flour
600ml (1 pint) skimmed milk from allowance
½ chicken stock cube

Cook the carrots, swede and potatoes in boiling salted water. Drain well. Place the carrots and swede in an ovenproof dish. Add the leeks, sweetcorn and tomatoes.

To make the sauce, mix the flour with a little of the milk until it forms a paste. Gradually add more milk, whisking all the time with a balloon whisk until all the milk is added. Place in a saucepan, add the stock cube and bring to the boil over a moderate heat, whisking all the time, and cook for 2–3 minutes to thicken.

Pour the white sauce over the vegetables in the ovenproof dish. Arrange the potatoes on top and sprinkle the mixed herbs and crushed cardamom over the top.

Mix the stuffing mix with the cheese and sprinkle on top.

Bake in a preheated oven at 190C, 375F or Gas Mark 5 for approximately 30 minutes until golden brown.

Serve with a green salad.

Vegetarian Chilli

SERVES 6

175g (6oz) [dry weight] rice
2 large onions, chopped
450g (1lb) mushrooms, chopped
425g (15oz) baked beans
1 x 400g (14oz) can Sainsbury's Kidney Beans in
Chilli Sauce
1 x 425g (15oz) can butter beans, drained
1 x 400g (14oz) can chopped tomatoes
2 teaspoons tomato purée

Boil the rice. When cooked drain well.

Dry-fry the onions and mushrooms in a non-stick pan for 5 minutes.

Add the baked beans, kidney beans, butter beans and tomatoes to the onion and mushroom mixture and heat slowly. Add the tomato purée and stir well until heated through.

When hot, serve the bean mixture with the rice.

Vegetable and Couscous Bake

SERVES 1

50g (2oz) easy-cook couscous
½ small onion, chopped
50g (2oz) carrots, sliced
25g (1oz) frozen peas
25g (1oz) frozen sweetcorn
50g (2oz) red kidney beans, drained
1 x 200g (7oz) can chopped tomatoes
2 teaspoons tomato purée
1 teaspoon garlic purée
1 level teaspoon mild chilli powder
2 teaspoons Worcester sauce
salt and pepper
1 Italian flavour stock cube

Pour 120ml (4fl oz) of boiling water over the couscous and cover for a few minutes until absorbed.

Soften the chopped onion in a little water in a microwave or dry-fry in a non-stick pan.

Boil the carrots in a saucepan until tender. Add the frozen vegetables for a few minutes.

Place the couscous in a casserole dish. Add the cooked vegetables, the red kidney beans and the chopped tomatoes. Mix in the tomato purée and garlic purée, chilli powder, Worcester sauce and seasoning.

Dissolve the stock cube in 150ml (¼ pint) of boiling water and stir into the mixture. Cover and cook in a preheated oven at 180C, 350F or Gas Mark 4 for 20–30 minutes. Check from time to time to make sure it does not dry out, and add a little water if necessary.

Serve with 115g (4oz) baby new potatoes.

Side Dishes

Fat-free Fluffy Rice

SERVES 8

450g (1lb) long-grain or Basmati rice
1 heaped teaspoon salt
4 or 5 cardamom seeds (optional)
½ teaspoon turmeric (optional)

Rinse the rice and place in a large non-stick pan. Fill with cold water. Add the salt and the cardamom seeds and turmeric (if using). Bring to the boil, stirring occasionally to prevent the rice from clumping, and simmer rapidly for 10–12 minutes.

Place the rice in a colander and rinse well under the cold tap until the residue salt has been washed away.

Return the rice to the pan, cover with a lid and leave on a very low heat for at least half an hour, turning the rice cccasionally with a non-scratch spoon to aid cooking. The rice will be ready when it is fluffy and soft to bite. If not quite cooked, add a tablespoon of water, stir, then replace the lid and cook a little longer. Remove the cardamom seeds (if using) before serving.

Dry-roast Potatoes

SERVES 3

450g (1lb) medium potatoes
1 vegetable or chicken stock cube
salt (optional)

Peel the potatoes. Bring a pan of water to the boil and add the stock cube.

Blanch the potatoes in the water for a few minutes.

Drain well and place on a baking tray. Lightly scratch the surface of each potato with a fork and sprinkle lightly with salt, if desired. Cook in a pre-heated oven at 200C, 400F or Gas Mark 6 for about 1 hour.

Garlic Potatoes

SERVES 4

450g (1lb) new potatoes
salt and pepper
1 medium onion, finely chopped
1 teaspoon plain flour
3 garlic cloves, crushed, or
1 teaspoon garlic granules
1 teaspoon mixed herbs
250ml (8fl oz) skimmed milk

Cook the potatoes in boiling salted water. Drain and leave to cool. Slice the cooked potatoes and arrange in layers in an ovenproof dish. Season well with salt and plenty of pepper.

Lightly dry-fry the onion in a non-stick pan until soft but not brown. Sprinkle carefully with flour. Add the garlic and herbs and stir well. Add the milk and cook over a low heat for 2–3 minutes.

Pour the mixture over the potatoes. Bake in a preheated oven at 180C, 350F or Gas Mark 4 for 30 minutes.

Dry-Fried Mushrooms

SERVES 4

450g (1lb) mushrooms
2 garlic cloves, crushed (optional)
salt and pepper

Cut the mushrooms in half and place in a non-stick pan. Add the garlic (if using), season with salt and pepper and dry-fry for about 5 minutes, stirring occasionally.

Transfer to an ovenproof dish. Cover and place in a preheated oven at 180C, 350F or Gas Mark 4 for 10 minutes.

Broad Bean and Mint Salad

SERVES 2–3

225g (8oz) shelled broad beans
150g (5oz) low-fat natural yogurt
1 tablespoon chopped fresh mint or to taste
1 teaspoon sugar
salt and pepper to taste
shredded lettuce

Cook the broad beans in a pan of boiling salted water for 10–15 minutes. Strain and allow to cool.

Mix the yogurt in a bowl with 1–2 tablespoons of cold water to the thickness you like your sauce.

Chop the fresh mint by adding 1 teaspoon of sugar on the top and then chopping it finely with a sharp knife or chopper. Add the mint to the yogurt and season with salt and pepper. Add the broad beans and stir well.

Arrange the shredded lettuce in a serving bowl and pour the broad bean mixture over the top. Serve well chilled.

Fire 'n' Ice Salad

SERVES 4

4 tomatoes, sliced
1 onion, sliced
120ml (4fl oz) white wine vinegar
1 teaspoon celery seeds
$\frac{1}{2}$ teaspoon dry mustard
large pinch of cayenne pepper
salt and freshly ground pepper
1 tablespoon sugar
4 ice cubes
8 strawberries (optional)

Place the tomatoes and onion in alternate layers in a deep bowl.

Combine the vinegar, celery seeds, mustard, cayenne pepper, salt and pepper and sugar in a small saucepan and boil for 1 minute. Pour over the onion

and tomatoes. Add the ice cubes and chill for at least
1 hour.

Drain the tomato and onion mixture, then spoon
into 4 individual dishes. Garnish with the strawberries (if using) and serve.

Pinto Bean Salad

SERVES 4

1 x 425g (15oz) can pinto beans
1 red grapefruit, broken into segments
1 medium red onion, finely chopped
Lesieur Fat Free French Dressing

Rinse the beans well under cold water. Cut the grapefruit segments into 1cm (½ inch) pieces.

Mix together the beans, grapefruit and onion, and
coat with the French dressing.

Chill for about 3 hours before serving.

Dressings

Fromage Frais Dressing

SERVES 1

3 tablespoons virtually fat-free fromage frais
3 pinches garam masala
½ teaspoon cumin seeds

Mix all the ingredients together and chill for 2 hours
before serving.

Oil-free Vinaigrette Dressing

3 tablespoons white wine vinegar or cider vinegar
1 tablespoon lemon juice
1½ teaspoons black pepper
½ teaspoon salt
1 teaspoon sugar
½ teaspoon French mustard
chopped herbs to taste (thyme,
marjoram, basil or parsley)

Place all the ingredients in a screw-top jar or container. Seal and shake well. Taste and add more salt or sugar as desired. Keep in the refrigerator and use within 3 days.

Citrus Dressing

120ml (4fl oz) fresh orange juice
50ml (2fl oz) lemon juice
50ml (2fl oz) wine vinegar
1 teaspoon Dijon mustard
salt and pepper

Place all the ingredients in a screw-top jar or container. Seal and shake well. Keep in the refrigerator and use within 3 days.

Desserts

Low-fat Chocolate Surprise Pudding

SERVES 8

3 large eggs, separated
75g (3oz) caster sugar
25g (1oz) chocolate icing sugar
115g (4oz) self-raising flour
50g (2oz) cornflour
2 tablespoons black cherry jam
1 large baking apple, peeled, cored and sliced

Whisk the egg whites until stiff. Add the yolks and whisk in.

Add the caster sugar and whisk, adding the icing sugar as you whisk, until all the sugar has dissolved.

Sift the self-raising flour with the cornflour. Fold half the flour into the egg and sugar mixture in a figure of eight action. When the flour is almost folded in, add the rest of the flour in the same way until the mixture is smooth. Set to one side.

Spoon the jam on the base of a lightly greased casserole dish. Place slices of apple in a spiral shape on top and place the remainder in the centre. Spoon the sponge mixture over the top.

Bake in a preheated oven at 180C, 350F or Gas Mark 4 for approximately 40 minutes or until golden brown.

Leave to cool for a few minutes, then loosen with a palette knife and turn out onto a flat dish. Serve with low-fat custard (allow 50ml/2fl oz per person).

Crunchy Plum Crumble

SERVES 4–6

450g (1lb) fresh plums or 1 large can plums
in natural juice, drained
½ tablespoon sugar (optional)
1 medium can peaches in natural juice, drained
1 teaspoon raisins
50g (2oz) cornflakes
50g (2oz) porridge oats
½ teaspoon ground cinnamon

If using fresh plums, stew them in a little water with the sugar.

Place the plums and peaches into a deep oven-proof dish. Add the raisins.

Crush the cornflakes and mix with the porridge oats, then sprinkle over the fruit. Sprinkle the cinnamon on top.

Bake in a preheated oven at 190C, 375F or Gas Mark 5 for 15 minutes.

Serve with low-fat custard (50ml/2fl oz per person).

Honey and Spice Pudding

SERVES 3–4

1 x 400g (14oz) can pears in natural juice, drained
2 eggs
25g (1oz) brown sugar
25g (1oz) clear honey
50g (2oz) self-raising flour
½ teaspoon mixed spice

Place the pears in an ovenproof dish.

Whisk together the eggs and sugar, then add the honey until the mixture is thick and creamy.

Sift the flour, then fold the flour and spice into the egg and honey mixture. Pour the mixture over the pears.

Bake in a preheated oven at 180C, 350F or Gas Mark 4 for approximately 40 minutes until golden brown.

Serve with low-fat custard (50ml/2fl oz per person) or very-low-fat fromage frais (50g/2oz per person).

Cranberry Pumpkin

SERVES 4–6

½ cup raw fresh or frozen cranberries
675g (1½lb) pumpkin, chopped
1 small apple, chopped
¼ cup chopped raisins
grated zest and juice of 1 orange
1½ tablespoons honey
dash of salt

Defrost the frozen cranberries (if using). Place the cranberries, pumpkin, apple and raisins in an oven-proof dish. Pour the juice and grated orange peel, and the honey and salt over the fruit.

Cover and bake in a preheated oven at 180C, 350F or Gas Mark 4 for 25–45 minutes.

Meringue Delight

SERVES 3–4

1 x 425g (14oz) can apricots in natural juice, drained
600ml (1 pint) very thick low-fat custard
made with custard powder and left to cool
whites of 2 large eggs
115g (4oz) caster sugar

Arrange the apricots on the base of an ovenproof dish. Pour the custard over.

Whisk the egg whites until stiff, then gradually add the caster sugar. Swirl this mixture over the custard.

Bake in a preheated oven at 190C, 375F or Gas Mark 5 for 10 minutes or until light golden.

Serve hot or cold.

Coffee and Banana Meringue

SERVES 6

for the meringue base
egg whites from 2 large eggs
1 tablespoon instant coffee powder
115g (4oz) caster sugar

for the topping
2 bananas
lemon juice
1 large scoop Wall's 'Too Good To Be True' vanilla
frozen dessert

To make the meringue base, whisk the egg whites and coffee powder until very stiff. Add 2 tablespoons of the sugar and whisk again until stiff. Fold in the remaining sugar.

Spread the mixture on non-stick (silicone) paper on a baking sheet to form a 20cm (8 inch) circle. Bake in the centre of a cool oven (190C, 225F or Gas Mark ¼) for about 4 hours.

Leave to cool and store in an airtight tin until required (the meringue will keep for about 2 weeks).

Just before serving, slice the bananas and toss in the lemon juice. Scoop the vanilla dessert onto the meringue base and arrange the bananas on top.

Low-fat Fruity Bread Pudding

SERVES 4

75g (3oz) mixed dried fruit
150ml (¼ pint) apple juice
115g (4oz) diced stale brown bread
1–1½ teaspoons cinnamon powder or
mixed spice
1 large banana, sliced
150ml (¼ pint) skimmed milk from allowance
1 tablespoon demerara sugar

Place the dried fruit and apple juice into a small pan. Bring to the boil and remove from the heat.

Stir the bread, spice or cinnamon and the banana into the fruit. Spoon into a shallow ovenproof dish. Pour the milk over the mixture and sprinkle the sugar on top.

Bake in a preheated oven at 200C, 400F or Gas Mark 6 for 25–30 minutes until golden brown.

Serve hot or cold with low-fat custard (50ml/2fl oz per person).

Rhubarb and Blackcurrant Jelly

SERVES 4

450g (1lb) rhubarb
600ml (1 pint) low-sugar blackcurrant Ribena
25g (1oz) gelatine or sugar-free jelly

Cut the rhubarb into 1cm (½ inch) pieces and simmer in 150ml (¼ pint) of the blackcurrant liquid until soft.

Heat the rest of the blackcurrant liquid until hot, then dissolve the gelatine or sugar-free jelly in it. Stir into the rhubarb. Leave to cool, then refrigerate until set.

Serve with low-fat fromage frais or low-fat natural yogurt (50ml/2fl oz per person).

Rhubarb Jelly

SERVES 3

450g (1lb) rhubarb
1 packet sugar-free jelly

Cook the rhubarb in 300ml (½ pint) water until it forms a pulp.

Beat with a wooden spoon or whisk until all the lumps have disappeared. Leave to cool.

Make up the jelly according to the instructions. Add to the rhubarb.

Pour into 3 sundae dishes and leave to set.

Chocolate Mousse

SERVES 4

1 x 215g (7½oz) carton Carnation Light
2 teaspoons powdered gelatine
1 sachet Ovaltine Options Choc-Orange or
Choc-O-Lait
mandarin segments to decorate

Chill the milk overnight in the refrigerator.

Sprinkle the gelatine onto 2 tablespoons of cold water in a cup and leave to stand for 5 minutes.

Stand the cup in a pan containing a little simmering water until the gelatine has dissolved.

Mix the Options with 2 tablespoons of hot water to a smooth paste. Add the gelatine and mix well.

Whip the milk until very frothy. Continue whipping as you add the gelatine and chocolate mixture.

Turn into a serving dish or 4 small dishes. Chill until set, then decorate with the mandarin segments.

Raspberry Mousse

SERVES 1

150ml (¼ pint) low-fat natural yogurt
15g (½oz) skimmed milk powder
2 teaspoons gelatine dissolved in
1 tablespoon hot water
115g (4oz) raspberries
artificial sweetener to taste

Place the yogurt, milk powder and gelatine in a blender and whiz for 30 seconds.

Add the raspberries and sweetener and blend again.

Pour into a dish and refrigerate for 1 hour.

Mango and Yogurt Mousse

SERVES 4–5

Fresh mangoes can be used in this recipe instead of canned ones. You will need two, weighing about 225g (8oz) each. Any canned fruit can be used instead of mango, but make sure it is canned in natural juice.

1 x 15g (½oz) packet powdered gelatine
1 x 275g (10oz) can mangoes
1 tablespoon lemon juice
300ml (½ pint) low-fat natural yogurt or
fromage frais
a little caster sugar or
artificial sweetener to taste (optional)
2 egg whites

Place 2 tablespoons of water in a small microwave or heatproof bowl and sprinkle the gelatine over. Dissolve the gelatine either by placing the bowl over a small pan of boiling water or placing it in the microwave on High for about 30 seconds or until dissolved.

Drain the mangoes and discard any syrup. Purée the mango flesh and lemon juice in a liquidiser, food processor or through a fine vegetable mill. Stir in the dissolved gelatine and leave until the mixture is just starting to set.

Fold in the yogurt or fromage frais. Taste and add a little sugar or artificial sweetener, if desired.

Whisk the egg whites until they are stiff and fold them carefully into the mixture. Pour the mixture into a wetted 600ml (1 pint) mould or pour into individual moulds. Chill overnight. Turn out and serve.

Mango Sorbet

SERVES 4–6

If you can't find large mangoes, use 4 smaller ones – you will need about 300ml (½ pint) of purée.

150g (5oz) granulated sugar
1 tablespoon lemon juice
2 large mangoes
1 large egg white
sprigs of mint to decorate

The sorbet will need to be frozen. If you will be using the freezing compartment of your refrigerator, turn it to the coldest setting about an hour before you start.

Place the sugar in a heavy-based pan with 300ml (½ pint) water and stir over a gentle heat until the sugar has dissolved. Bring to the boil and boil for 5 minutes without stirring. Allow to cool until tepid.

Cut the mangoes in half and scoop out the flesh with a metal spoon. Reserve the mango skins. Purée the flesh with a little of the syrup in a liquidiser, food processor or vegetable mill. Stir into the syrup and leave until completely cold.

Sieve the mixture through a fine strainer and pour into a freezer-proof dish. Cover and place in the freezer for about an hour until the mixture has frozen to the depth of 2.5cm (1 inch) around the sides of the container.

At this stage, turn the mixture into a bowl and whisk well with a fork or electric whisk until the mixture is quite smooth and without ice crystals. Return to the freezer compartment, cover and freeze again for a further 30 minutes.

Turn the mixture into a bowl and whisk again until smooth.

Whisk the egg white until it stands in soft peaks, and fold into the ice mixture. Return to the freezer compartment again and leave for several hours or until required.

Half an hour before serving place the sorbet in the refrigerator. To serve, spoon the sorbet into the reserved mango skins or in individual glasses and decorate with sprigs of mint.

Chestnut Sundae

SERVES 4

75g (3oz) unsweetened chestnut purée
2 tablespoons low-fat natural yogurt
600ml (1 pint) low-fat vanilla ice cream
2 meringues, crushed

Mix the chestnut purée and yogurt together in a bowl.

Place scoops of the ice cream into individual serving dishes. Sprinkle the crushed meringue over the top, and top with the chestnut mixture.

Morello Cherries and Melon Balls

SERVES 4

115g (4oz) caster sugar
1 x 1cm (½ inch) piece cinnamon
zest of 1 orange, lemon or lime
450g (1lb) morello cherries
1 melon

Place the sugar, cinnamon and zest into a pan. Add 150ml (¼ pint) water, bring to the boil and simmer for a few minutes.

Add the cherries and bring back to the boil, then reduce the heat and poach until the cherry stems soften.

Remove the cherries and place into a bowl.

Reduce the syrup until it thickens, then pour it over the cherries (including the cinnamon).

Leave to cool, then refrigerate.

Halve the melon and use a melon-cutter to cut out balls from the melon flesh.

Serve the cherries and syrup with the melon balls.

Apple and Orange Dessert

SERVES 6

6 dessert apples
250ml (8fl oz) diet lemonade
3 oranges
50g (2oz) caster sugar

Peel, core and quarter the apples and poach gently in the diet lemonade. Leave to cool.

Using a potato peeler, peel half of one orange and cut the peel into thin strips. Boil this in a little water for 5 minutes.

Strain and rinse under cold water.

To make the caramel, place the caster sugar in a pan with a little water. Heat gently to dissolve the sugar, then boil again quickly until the sugar turns golden. Pour into a non-stick baking tin and leave to set. When set, break up into small pieces.

Cut the oranges into segments and place in a serving dish. Add the apples and a little of the juice. Sprinkle the caramel bits and orange peel strips over and serve with low-fat fromage frais (50g/2oz per person).

Apple, Orange and Pineapple Bake

SERVES 4

2 oranges
4 baking apples
2 teaspoons brown sugar
4 pineapple rings
50g (2oz) Grape Nuts cereal
50g (2oz) oat flakes
1 teaspoon ground cinnamon
1 teaspoon ground cloves
120ml (4fl oz) pineapple juice

Grate the zest from the oranges and break the oranges into segments. Chop the segments.

Peel and core the apples and cut into quarters.

Sprinkle the sugar over the bottom of a baking dish. Arrange the pineapple rings in the dish, then arrange the apples on top.

Sprinkle the chopped orange segments over the apple and pineapple mixture.

Mix the Grape Nuts, orange zest, oat flakes, cinnamon and cloves in a bowl and spread over the mixture. Drizzle the pineapple juice over the dry mixture.

Bake in a preheated oven at 180C, 350F or Gas Mark 4 for 30 minutes. Serve hot.

Fruit Fool

SERVES 4–6

1 packet sugar-free jelly
115g (4oz) fresh fruit (soft fruit is best, e.g.
strawberries, raspberries, blackcurrants)
artificial sweetener (optional)
225g (8oz) very-low-fat fromage frais

Make up the jelly with 150ml (¼ pint) boiling water.

Sprinkle a little artificial sweetener on the fruit if desired. Stir the fruit into the jelly and make up to 450ml (¾ pint) with cold water. Place in the refrigerator until nearly set.

When the jelly is almost set, stir in the fromage frais and whisk until light and fluffy. Chill thoroughly before serving.

RECIPES

Baked Nectarines

SERVES 2–4

2 nectarines
1 tablespoon honey
4 heaped tablespoons muesli
2 teaspoons dark brown sugar

Cut the nectarines in half and remove the stones. Place the nectarines, cut-side down, under a medium grill for a few minutes.

Turn them over and remove the skin, then grill for a further 5 minutes.

Spread the cut-side with the honey and grill for 3 minutes.

Mix the muesli with sugar, then spoon onto the nectarines and replace under the heat for a further 3 minutes.

Serve with low-fat yogurt (50g/2oz per person).

Peach Pud

SERVES 4

For a special occasion, you can leave out the lemon juice in this recipe and substitute 1 tablespoon of brandy.

1 large can peaches
1 small pot natural set low-fat yogurt
1 tablespoon lemon juice
1 teaspoon vanilla essence
1 large can low-fat custard
mixed spice to decorate

Drain the peaches and place in a food processor or liquidiser. Add the yogurt and purée until smooth. Alternatively, pass the peaches through a vegetable mill and then stir in the yogurt.

Mix the lemon juice and vanilla essence with the custard.

Fold the custard mixture into the puréed peaches and yogurt.

To serve, pour into 4 glasses and decorate with a shake of mixed spice.

Grapefruit and Yogurt Delight

SERVES 2–3

220g (7½oz) canned grapefruit in natural juice
Canderel Spoonful or similar
1 x 150g (5oz) carton very-low-fat yogurt or
fromage frais
1 packet low-fat Horlicks powder

Divide the grapefruit and juice into 2 or 3 fruit glasses. Sprinkle quite liberally with the Canderel Spoonful to taste. Top with the yogurt or fromage frais and sprinkle the Horlicks powder over the top.

Grapefruit Wobble

SERVES 6

1 sachet gelatine
150ml (¼ pint) orange juice
1 x 539 g (1lb 6oz) can grapefruit segments
in natural juice
1 orange, cut into thin slices

Dissolve the gelatine in a little of the orange juice over a pan of hot water or in a microwave.

Drain the juice from the can of grapefruit, add the rest of the orange juice and make up to 450ml (¾ pint). Add the dissolved gelatine and mix well, then stir in the grapefruit segments. Leave to set.

When set, chop up roughly, place into individual glasses and decorate with whole or halved slices of orange.

Low-fat Trifle

SERVES 4

1 packet sugar-free jelly
1 jam Swiss roll
1 x 400g (14oz) can any fruit in natural juice
1 packet low-fat instant custard

Make up the jelly according to the directions, using the juice from the canned fruit.

Cut up the Swiss roll and place in a large dish. Add the drained fruit, cover with the jelly and leave to set.

Make up the custard using just under the amount of water instructed. Leave to cool.

When the jelly is set, cover with the cool custard and leave to set.

Serve with low-fat fromage frais (50g/2oz per person).

Spiced Tropical Fruit Salad

SERVES 4

2 limes
½ medium melon, chopped
1 ripe mango, chopped
2 kiwi fruits, sliced
½ small ripe pineapple, cut into chunks
1 orange, broken into segments
2 bananas, sliced
1 star fruit, sliced

for the syrup
1–2 small chillies
50g (2oz) sugar or artificial sweetener to taste

To make the syrup, deseed and chop the chillies finely. Dissolve the sugar in 350ml (12fl oz) water and boil for 5 minutes. Add the chopped chillies. Taste frequently and remove the chillies when the syrup seems hot enough.

Using a potato peeler, thinly pare off the zest of 1 lime, cut into fine shreds and blanch for 5–10 minutes in boiling water. Drain and refresh under cold water.

Place the fruit in a bowl. Add the lime shreds and juice of the 2 limes, then pour the chilli syrup over the fruit. Refrigerate for ½–1 hour before serving.

Summer Fruit Salad

SERVES 4

115g (4oz) black grapes
115g (4oz) seedless green grapes
115g (4oz) strawberries
2–3 small tangerines
½ honeydew melon, peeled
1 large crisp eating apple
2–3 tablespoons lemon juice
300ml (½ pint) orange or apple juice
artificial sweetener to taste

Cut the black grapes in half and remove the seeds. Leave the green grapes whole. Hull and slice the strawberries. Peel the tangerines and break into segments. Peel the melon, remove the seeds and slice the flesh. Peel, core and slice the apple.

Mix all the fruit together and stir in the lemon juice, making sure that the apple is well coated. Pour the orange juice or apple juice over the fruit and mix well. Sweeten to taste with the artificial sweetener.

Place in a bowl, cover with lid or cling film, and chill in the refrigerator for at least an hour before serving.

Banana Cream Topping

SERVES 4

This is a delicious topping to use on any cold fruit, and because it is quite sweet the fruit does not need to be sweetened.

1 egg white
1 ripe banana, mashed
50g (2oz) caster sugar
pinch of salt
1 teaspoon lemon juice

Whisk the egg white, then whisk in all the remaining ingredients. Chill and serve the same day.

Snacks

Not Naughty But Nice Strawberry Whip

SERVES 1

1 cup skimmed milk from allowance
4 large strawberries, hulled, or
2 teaspoons strawberry jam

Place the cup of milk in the freezer for an hour until crystals form.

When the milk is ready, place it in a food processor or whip it into cream. Add the strawberries or jam to the mixture and give them a quick burst. Eat immediately.

Cool and Refreshing Yogurt Drink

MAKES APPROX. 1.2 LITRES (2 PINTS)

500g (1¼lb) very-low-fat yogurt or fromage frais
¼–½ cucumber, finely chopped
salt

In a mixing bowl, blend the yogurt or fromage frais with the chopped cucumber. Add cold water until the mixture resembles milk. Add salt to taste. Keep refrigerated.

Strawberry Muffins

MAKES 10 MUFFINS

40g (1½oz) Tesco 95% Fat Free Sunflower Spread
225g (8oz) wholemeal self-raising flour
40g (1½oz) brown sugar
1 x 410g (14oz) can strawberries in light juice
1 egg, beaten

Rub the sunflower spread into the flour, add the brown sugar and stir well.

Drain the strawberries and reserve the juice.

Slightly mash the strawberries so that they are no longer whole, and stir into the flour mixture. Add 7 tablespoons of strawberry juice, then add the beaten egg and stir well.

Spoon the mixture into 10 deep muffin cases. Bake in the centre of a preheated oven at 180C, 350F or Gas Mark 4 for 25 minutes.

Store in an airtight tin for 24 hours before serving.

Apple and Sultana Cake

1 X 1CM (½ INCH) SLICE PER SERVING

1 cup All-Bran cereal
½ cup skimmed or semi-skimmed milk
75g (3oz) sultanas
1 cup sugar
1 cup self-raising flour
1 cup grated cooking apple (about 2–3 apples)
1 heaped teaspoon ground cinnamon

Place the All-Bran cereal in the milk, add the sultanas and sugar and leave to soak for about 30 minutes.

Add the grated apple to the mixture and stir in the self-raising flour and the cinnamon.

Place the mixture in a baking tin lined with grease-proof paper and bake in a preheated oven at 150C, 300F or Gas Mark 2 for 1½–2 hours. To check if the cake is cooked, insert a skewer in the centre of the cake. If the skewer comes out clean, the cake is cooked.

Leave to cool in the tin. When cold wrap in grease-proof paper and tin foil.

Spicy Apple Cake

1 X 1CM (½ INCH) SLICE PER SERVING

225g (8oz) wholemeal self-raising flour
75g (3oz) light brown sugar
2 teaspoons cinnamon
175g (6oz) sultanas
1 baking apple
250ml (8fl oz) skimmed milk

Mix together the flour, sugar and cinnamon. Add the sultanas and stir well.

Peel, core and grate the apple and add to the mixture. Add the milk and stir well.

Place the mixture in a lined 20 x 13cm (8 x 5in) loaf tin or a 15cm (6 inch) round cake tin. Bake in the centre of a preheated oven at 160C, 325F or Gas Mark 3 for 1¼ hours. Leave to cool in the tin.

Coffee and Orange Slab

1 X 1CM (½ INCH) SLICE PER SERVING

375g (13oz) self-raising flour
150g (5oz) caster sugar
½ teaspoon salt
1½ teaspoons baking powder
½ teaspoon bicarbonate of soda
2 tablespoons coffee blended with
hot water to dissolve
25g (1oz) polyunsaturated margarine
1 egg, beaten
350–375ml (12–13fl oz) skimmed milk
icing sugar or ground ginger to decorate

Sift all the dry ingredients together, add the blended coffee and mix well.

Melt the margarine. Make a well in the centre of the mixture and add the melted margarine and the beaten egg. Add the milk, adding sufficient milk until the mixture is sloppy but holds its shape. Stir well.

Place the mixture into a lined Swiss roll tin and bake in a preheated oven at 180C, 350F or Gas Mark 4 for 20–30 minutes or until firm to the touch.

Decorate with plain icing sugar mixed with water, or sprinkle ground ginger on top.

Malt Loaf

1 X 1CM (½ INCH) SLICE PER SERVING

2 tablespoons malt
2 tablespoons Golden Syrup
1 cup skimmed milk
225g (8oz) plain flour
75g (3oz) chopped dates or sultanas
1 egg, beaten
1 level teaspoon bicarbonate of soda

Place the malt, syrup and milk in a saucepan and heat until well blended.

Sieve the flour into a bowl and add the fruit. Stir the egg and the malt mixture into the flour and fruit.

Dissolve the bicarbonate of soda in a little water and add to the mixture.

Pour the mixture into a lined 450g (1lb) baking tin and bake in a preheated oven at 180C, 350F or Gas Mark 4 for about an hour until raised and golden.

When cooked, remove the tin from the oven and wrap the loaf in a cloth to keep the cake moist.

7

The New Body
Workout

New Body is a unique workout designed to reshape your body. It's safe and incredibly effective.

If we want to keep our heart and lungs in good condition and burn unwanted fat, we need to do regular aerobic exercise. And if we want to tighten and tone our bodies, we need to do toning exercises that work specific muscle groups. Toning exercises also help protect against the brittle bone disease osteoporosis. This New Body Workout integrates both these elements – making it doubly effective, yet saves you time!

To burn fat through exercise you need to increase your pulse rate. With this in mind, in my New Body Workout I have combined some low-impact aerobic moves with toning exercises to enable you to burn fat, increase your stamina and tone your muscles very effectively – all at the same time.

Aerobic exercise can also be taken in many other forms, such as brisk walking, skipping, running or swimming. After you have warmed up, as long as you are mildly out of breath, you will be achieving a fat-burning effect. Do not push yourself too hard, though, as to do so would switch your body's energy systems away from fat-burning and on to a system that draws on its carbohydrate stores. For maximum fat-burning benefits, aim for 20–30 minutes at a moderate pace, rather than short, sharp bursts. Try to make activity part of your everyday lifestyle, not just something you do while you're on your weight-reducing diet.

How to use the New Body Workout to best effect

This New Body Workout is divided into six 10-minute sections, each of which targets a specific area of the body – hips and thighs, upper arms, chest and upper back, abdominals and back, upper body, lower body – so that you can design your own workout and concentrate on those areas that require particular attention. But there's nothing to stop you doing all six sections so that you see and feel the benefits all over.

All the standing exercises are fat-burning, as they incorporate general bodily movements designed to elevate the heart rate. The exercises performed sitting or lying on the floor work specific muscle groups and should be attempted regularly to achieve maximum benefits to your shape and muscle tone. A combination of both aerobic and toning moves is the ideal.

Some of the exercises incorporate the use of handweights, which can really help speed up the reshaping process. However, I suggest you start out without the handweights and familiarise yourself with the moves. Then, as you become stronger, you can progress by adding the handweights. You should find a selection of handweights at your local sports shop. Make sure they are comfortable to hold and choose between 0.5kg and 1kg weights. Alternatively, you can make your own by filling two plastic bottles with water or sand or use cans of beans. When using weights, keep your wrists firm and try not to grip the weights too tightly. If you prefer not to use handweights, don't worry. Using your own body weight for resistance will still be effective.

Guidelines are given for repetitions, but don't worry if you can't do all the suggested repetitions at first. Just build up slowly and begin with a few repetitions and gradually increase the number each time you work out. Working a muscle too hard too soon runs the risk of damaging the muscle. Although each exercise should cause some mild discomfort in order to provide sufficient challenge, you should not feel any pain.

Each time you work out, always start with the warm-up moves on pages 199–203, followed by the preparatory stretches on pages 203–205, then add on your selected toning routine(s). Finish with the cool-down stretches on pages 230–235 to enable your muscles to return to normal and prevent any aches or pains later.

Aim to do these exercises at least three days a week, since consistency is important if you are to see results. The more often you do them, the faster your progress will be. However, you should always have one rest day from exercise each week, so decide which day this will be and, although you can still be active, it's a good idea not to challenge your body on this day.

The New Body Workout

Warming Up
Preparatory Stretches
Section One: Hips and Thighs
Section Two: Upper Arms
Section Three: Chest and Upper Back
Section Four: Abdominals and Back
Section Five: Upper Body
Section Six: Lower Body
Cool-down Stretches

Warming Up

1 HEEL DIGS

Do alternate heel digs in front, while simultaneously pushing your arms out forwards at shoulder level. Keep your shoulders back and down and your tummy tight. Repeat 16 times.

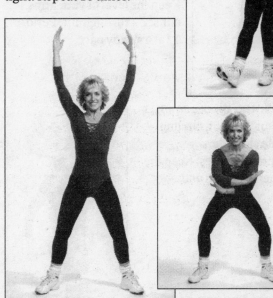

2 CIRCLING SQUATS

Stand with feet a comfortable distance apart. As you bend and straighten your legs, make a large circle with your arms. Stand tall throughout and control the arm movement. Repeat 12 times.

199

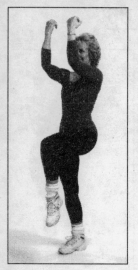

3 KNEE LIFTS WITH PEC DEC

Stand with feet slightly apart. Bring your arms out to the sides, with your elbows at shoulder height, and bend them at a 90-degree angle. As you lift alternate knees, bring your elbows close together in front of your chest, then open them out to the sides again. Keep the level of your arms constant throughout. Perform 12 at a steady pace.

4 MARCH AND SHOULDER ROLLS

March on the spot, circling alternate shoulders backwards 10 times. Keep the movement smooth and controlled.

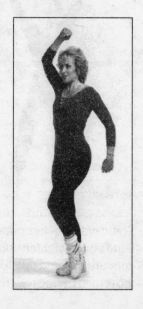

5 KNEE LIFTS

Lift alternate knees at a steady pace and bring the opposite hand to touch the raised knee. Repeat 16 times, keeping your back straight and your shoulders back and down.

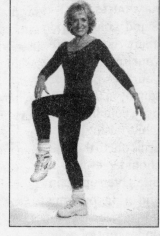

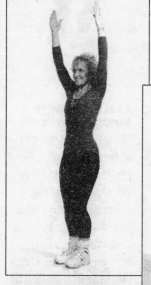

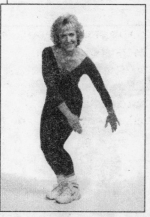

6 TWISTED SKI SWINGS

With feet together and tummy pulled in tight, lift both arms above your head. Now swing down to one side, bending your knees and keeping your back straight. Lift up and repeat on the other side. Repeat 8 times on each side.

7 KNEE BENDS WITH ARM RAISES

Stand with feet wide apart. As you bend your knees in line with your toes, pull your tummy in tight and push your hips back while raising both arms out to the sides at shoulder level. Straighten up again and bring your arms down. Repeat 10 times under control.

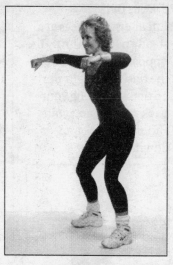

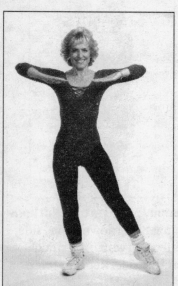

8 HALF JACKS WITH SHOULDER PRESS

With elbows bent at shoulder height, push one foot out to the side and at the same time press your shoulders back. Keep changing legs and repeat 16 times. Keep your tummy pulled in tight and control the move.

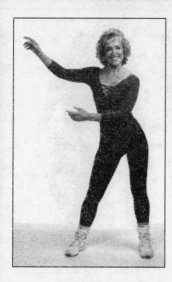

9 HIP SHIFTS

Stand with feet hip-width apart, knees slightly bent, tummy tight and back straight. Move your hips rhythmically from side to side while letting your arms move naturally in the opposite direction. Repeat 8 times.

Preparatory Stretches

1 INNER THIGH AND OBLIQUE STRETCH

Stand with feet wide apart. Keep your hips facing forwards, slightly turn out your left foot and aim your right foot forwards. Bend your left knee and feel the stretch in the inner thigh of your right leg. Place your left hand on your left thigh for support, reach your right arm up and lean towards the bent leg. Hold for 8 seconds. Repeat on the other side.

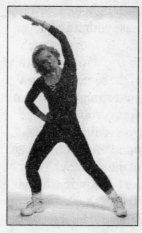

203

2 QUADRICEPS STRETCH

Stand on your right leg with your right knee slightly bent. Keep your tummy tight, your back straight and keep looking forwards. Bend your left leg behind you and hold onto the ankle with your left hand. Keep the knees level and ease the left hip forwards slightly. Hold for 8 seconds. Release and repeat with the other leg.

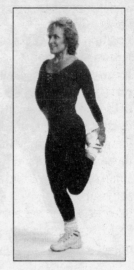

3 INNER THIGH AND SHOULDER STRETCH

Stand with feet wide apart. Keeping your hips facing forwards, slightly turn out your left foot and point your right foot forwards. Ease your weight over the left foot to stretch the right inner thigh and at the same time draw your straight right arm across your chest and press with the other hand to stretch the back of the shoulder. Hold for 8 seconds. Change to the other leg and arm and hold for 8 seconds.

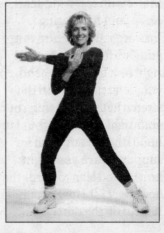

4 FRONT OF THIGH, HIP AND CHEST STRETCH

Position one foot behind you and bend both knees. Raise your back heel and rest your weight on the ball of the foot. Bend slightly deeper, pressing your hips forwards and at the same time place your hands in the small of your back and squeeze the shoulder blades together behind you. Hold for 8 seconds, then repeat with the other leg.

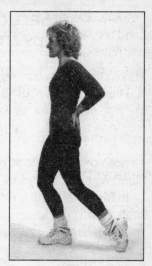

5 CALF AND TRICEPS STRETCH

Stand with feet slightly apart. Step well back with the left foot, keeping both feet facing forwards and both heels down. Bend your right knee over the toes and keep the left leg straight. Feel the stretch in the left calf. At the same time bend one arm back behind the shoulder and use the other hand to ease it further back. Feel the stretch in the

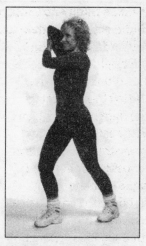

triceps (back of upper arm). Hold for 8 seconds, then change to the other arm and leg and hold for 8 seconds.

Section One:
Hips and Thighs

Make sure you warm up first (see page 199). When you have completed the hip and thigh exercises, if you are not moving on to another section, turn to the cool-down stretches on page 230 to finish.

1 FRONT OF THIGH AND BOTTOM TONER
Stand with feet hip-width apart and hands on hips. Lean forwards slightly with your weight on your heels. Bend your knees and at the same time push your hips back as if you were about to sit on a chair. Squeeze your bottom as you straighten up again. Repeat 10 times.

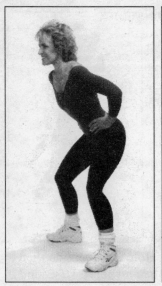 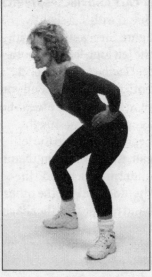

2 STANDING INNER THIGH TONER

Stand with hands on hips (or with one hand on a chair or wall for support) and lift one foot out to the side. Keeping your body upright and tummy pulled in tight, draw the 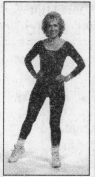 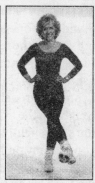 raised leg across the body, leading with the ankle. Take the leg out to the side again and repeat. Move slowly and under control, keeping the supporting leg slightly bent. Repeat 8 times, then repeat with the other leg.

3 STANDING THIGH AND BOTTOM TONER

Stand with one foot in front of the other, with the rear foot well back. Your weight should be evenly distributed between both legs. Maintaining an upright position, slowly lower your body down until both knees are at a 90-degree angle, then push up again slowly without fully extending the knees. Repeat 6 times, then change to the other leg in front and repeat.

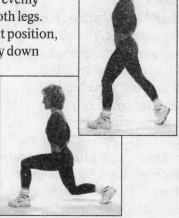

4 STANDING HAMSTRING TONER

Stand with one foot in front of the other, with the rear foot well back. Place your hands on your hips (or use a chair or wall for support). Lean forwards slightly with your weight on the front knee, keeping the knee slightly bent and your tummy pulled in tight. At the same time lift the back leg off the floor, bringing the heel towards your bottom. Bend and straighten the leg 8 times, then repeat with the other leg. Repeat the whole sequence again.

5 STANDING OUTER THIGH TONER

Stand with hands on hips (or use a chair or wall for support) and, maintaining an upright posture, place your weight firmly on your leg. Gently lift the non-weight-bearing leg out to the side to about 45 degrees, without tipping the upper body, then lower the leg and repeat. Repeat 8 times, then change and repeat with the other leg.

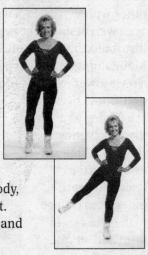

6 STANDING BOTTOM TONER

Stand with one foot in front of the other, with the rear foot well back. Place your hands on your hips (or use a chair or wall for support). Lean forwards slightly with your weight on the front foot, with the front knee slightly bent and tummy pulled in tight. At the same time lift the back leg off the floor, keeping the back leg straight and both hips facing forwards. Lift and lower the leg 8 times, squeezing your bottom as you lift. Do not lift too high. Repeat with the other leg, then repeat the whole sequence again.

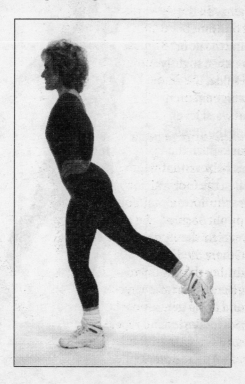

Section Two:
Upper Arms

If you are starting your workout with this section, warm up first (see page 199). After completing the upper arm exercises, move on to another section or turn to the cool-down stretches on page 230.

1 TRICEPS AND HIP TONER

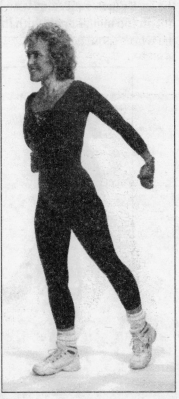

Stand with feet together, with the ball of one foot touching the floor and the knee slightly bent. Hold a handweight in each hand at waist level. Keeping the elbows well back, push the bent leg back so that the ball of the foot touches the floor behind you. As you do so, extend the arm on the same side to straighten the elbow. Bend the arm again and bring the foot back in. Repeat 8 times on one side, then repeat on the other side.

2 UNDERARM TONER

Stand with feet wide apart and hold a handweight in each hand. Bend one leg slightly and place the opposite hand behind your shoulder, using the other hand to support the arm. As you bend alternate legs, extend the arm up, without locking the elbow, and then bend it again. Keep your head upright and perform under control. Repeat 8 times, then change arms and repeat.

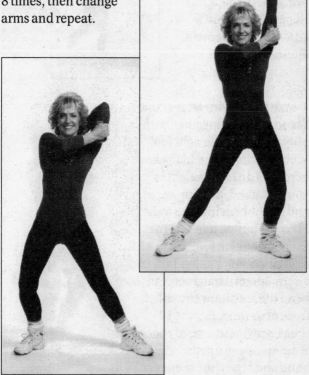

3 FOREARM PRESS

Stand with feet together, arms by your sides, and hold a handweight in each hand. Extend one leg behind and at the same time raise both arms in front to chest height. Keep your tummy pulled in tight and the front knee slightly bent, and try not to lean forwards. Lower the arms and bring the leg back in. Repeat 12 times in a controlled movement, alternating legs.

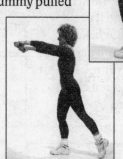

4 STEP TOUCH WITH BICEPS CURL

Stand with feet together, with only the ball of the right foot touching the floor and the knee bent. Hold a handweight in your left hand, palm upwards and elbow bent into the waist. Place your right hand on the front of your left forearm to add resistance. As you step-tap onto alternate feet, straighten and bend the left elbow to work the front of the arm. Repeat 12 times, moving at a steady pace. Place the weight in the right hand and repeat the sequence.

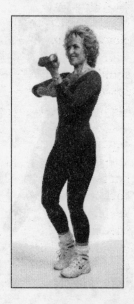

Section Three:
Chest and Upper Back

If you are starting your workout with this section, warm up first (see page 199). After completing the chest and upper back exercises, move on to another section or turn to the cool-down stretches on page 230.

1 POSTURE IMPROVER WITH KNEE BENDS

Stand with feet together and hold a handweight in each hand. Bring both arms up to chest height, with elbows in line with the shoulders, and smoothly press the shoulders back while bending your knees. Bend the knees and press back 6 times, keeping your head up and tummy pulled in tight throughout. Rest, then repeat.

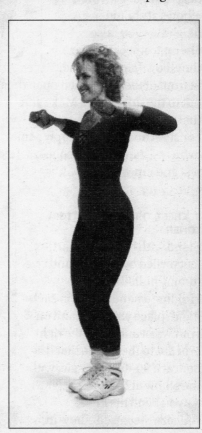

2 CHEST TONER WITH KNEE RAISES

Stand with feet together and hold a handweight in each hand. Bring your arms out to the sides so that they are bent at a 90-degree angle with the elbows at shoulder height. As you raise alternate knees, squeeze the elbows close together in front of the chest, then open them out to the sides again. Make sure that the level of the arms stays constant and that you apply some extra resistance as you squeeze. Repeat 8 times, then rest and repeat.

3 CHEST, THIGH AND BOTTOM TONER

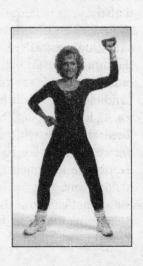

Stand with feet wide apart, feet turned out slightly and tummy pulled in tight. Holding a handweight in each hand, place your left hand on your waist and bring the right arm out to the side so that it is bent at a 90-degree angle, with the elbow at shoulder height. As you bend the knees, squeeze the raised elbow in

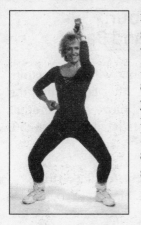

front of your chest, then straighten the knees and take the arm out to the side again. Make sure that the level of the arm stays constant and that you apply some extra resistance as you squeeze. Repeat 8 times, then change arms and repeat on the other side.

4 UPPER BACK TONER

Stand with feet apart, knees bent, and hold a handweight in each hand. Holding your tummy in tight to support your back, take your body weight forwards but make sure you are well balanced and bring your arms in front. Stay in this position as you ease the shoulders back, drawing the shoulder blades together behind you. Extend the arms forward again, then repeat the squeezing movement and concentrate on drawing the shoulder blades together. Repeat 8 times. Rest, then repeat.

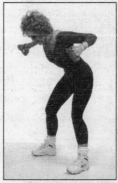

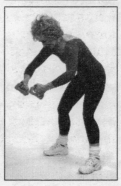

Section Four:
Abdominals and Back

If you are starting your workout with this section, warm up first (see page 199). After completing the abdominal and back exercises, move on to another section or turn to the cool-down stretches on page 230.

1 TUMMY TONER

Lie on your back, with knees bent, feet flat on the floor and tummy pulled in tight. Make sure your lower back is in contact with the floor. Place one hand to the side of your head and rest the other hand on your thigh. Slowly lift your upper body off the floor, and slide your hand towards your knee, then slowly lower to the floor again. Breathe out as you lift and breathe in as you lower, keeping your chin away from your chest. Repeat 8 times. Rest and repeat.

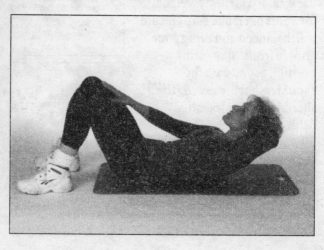

2 WAIST TONER

Lie on your back, with knees bent, feet flat on the floor and tummy pulled in tight. Place your left hand to the back of your head to support your neck. Slowly lift off the floor and rotate the upper body to the left, sliding your right arm in the direction of your left knee. Keep the left elbow on the floor for support. Slowly lower to the floor again. Repeat 6 times, breathing out as you lift and breathing in as you lower. Relax, then change arms and repeat the exercise to work the other side of the waist. Rest, then repeat the whole sequence once more.

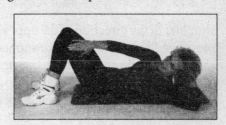

3 ADVANCED TUMMY CURL

Lie on your back, with knees bent, feet flat on the floor and tummy pulled in tight. Place your hands to either side of your head to support the neck. Slowly lift your upper body off the floor, keeping your chin away from your chest, and at the same time lift one foot off the floor slightly. Slowly lower to the floor again, and repeat, this time raising the other foot. Breathe out as you lift and breathe in as you lower. Repeat 8 times. Rest and repeat.

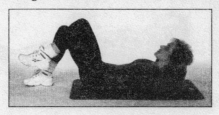

4 ADVANCED WAIST TRIMMER

Lie on your back, with knees bent, feet flat on the floor and tummy pulled in tight. Place your hands to

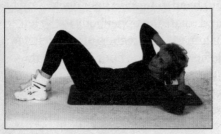

either side of your head to support the neck. Slowly lift your upper body off the floor and rotate one shoulder in the direction of the opposite knee. Keep the other elbow on the floor for support. Slowly lower to the floor again and repeat to the other side. Breathe out as you lift and breathe in as you lower, keeping your chin away from your chest. Repeat 12 times.

5 TUMMY FLATTENER

Lie on your front and rest your chin on your hands. Slowly and smoothly pull your abdominal muscles in tight, keeping your chest and thighs in contact with the floor. Hold for 8 seconds, breathing normally, then relax. Repeat twice more.

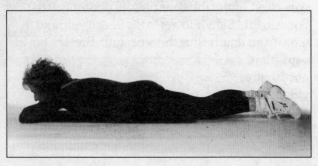

6 SPINE CONTROL

Come up into the all fours' position. Check that you are in a square position with your hands directly under your shoulders and your knees under your hips. Pull your tummy in tight to flatten the spine. Reach out and slowly lift the right arm and left leg off the floor, keeping the movement controlled. Release, then change sides to repeat with the other arm and leg. Breathe out as you reach and breathe in as you lower. Repeat 6 times, changing sides each time.

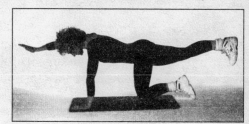

7 BACK STRENGTHENER

Lie on your front, with both arms extended in front and resting on the floor. Keep both hips facing the floor

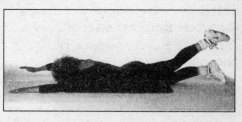

and your head facing down, slowly lift the right arm and left leg off the floor. Do not lift too high. Now lower the arm and leg to the floor and repeat with the left arm and right leg. Repeat 12 times (6 on each side).

8 BACK RAISES

Lie face down, with arms by your sides, palms facing upwards. Using only the strength in your back, slowly raise your head and shoulders off the floor, then lower them again. Repeat this small movement 6 times, moving slowly and under control. Rest, then repeat.

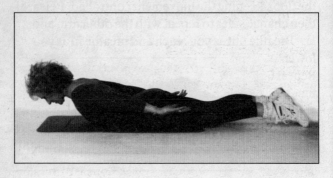

Section Five:
Upper Body

If you are starting your workout with this section, warm up first (see page 199). After completing the upper body exercises, move on to another section or turn to the cool-down stretches on page 230.

1 SHOULDER STRENGTHENER

Sit in a comfortable cross-legged position, with your back straight and tummy pulled in tight. Hold a handweight in each hand. Begin with your elbows bent close to your waist. Carefully lift the arms out to the sides to shoulder height, then lower them again, keeping the elbows bent throughout. Breathe out as you lift and breathe in as you lower. Repeat 8 times. Rest, then repeat if you can. This exercise can be done in the standing position if you prefer.

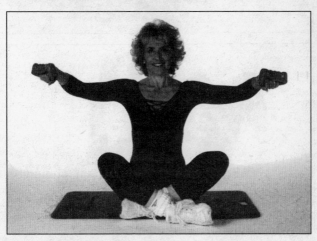

2 LYING CHEST TONER

Lie on your back, with both knees bent, and hold a handweight in each hand. Pull your tummy in tight and make sure your back is supported by the floor. Bring your arms out to the sides, with elbows bent at a 90-degree angle and level with your shoulders. Squeeze the bent arms towards each other in front of your chest, then open them out to the sides again. Exhale as the arms come in and breathe in as the arms move out. Repeat 8 times. Rest, then repeat if you can.

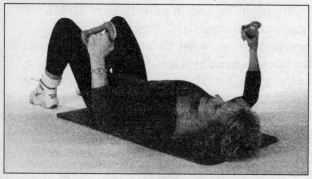

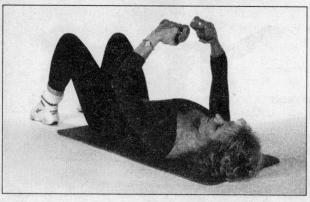

3 LYING UNDERARM TONER

Lie on your back, with knees bent and tummy pulled in tight. Hold a handweight in one hand and bring that hand close to your ear, with the elbow pointing towards the ceiling. Support the back of the arm with

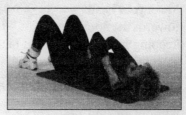

the other hand. Slowly and under control, extend your arm, without locking the elbow, then bend the arm back to the starting position. Breathe out as you extend the arm and breathe in as you lower it. Repeat 10 times. Rest, then repeat with the other arm.

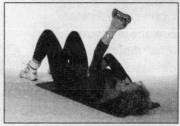

4 SEATED UPPER BACK TONER

Sit in a comfortable cross-legged position, with your back straight, tummy tight, and head facing forwards.

Place your hands on your shoulders. Maintaining a good posture, slowly draw the shoulder blades together, then release. Repeat 8 times slowly and under control. Rest, then repeat.

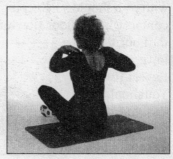

5 PRESS-UPS

Position yourself on your hands and knees, with your knees under your hips and your hands under your shoulders. Bend your elbows and lower your head towards the floor, keeping your forehead in front of your hands. Straighten up again, without locking the elbows, and repeat. Breathe in as you lower and breathe out as you lift. Do 8 press-ups under control. Rest, and repeat.

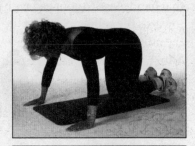

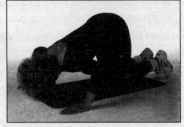

6 POSTURE IMPROVER

Lie face down. Bend both arms at a 90-degree angle and place them on the floor so that the elbows are level with your shoulders. Keeping your head and hips in contact with the floor, slowly raise your bent arms off the floor, then lower them again. Repeat 10 times. You should feel this working the middle of the upper back.

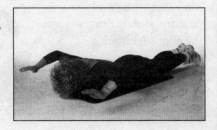

7 UNDERARM TONER

Kneel on your left leg and support your weight on your bent right leg, with your right arm resting on it. Holding a handweight in your left hand, bend your arm and place your left hand on your waist. Slowly straighten the arm behind you to work the tricep muscle at the back of the upper arm, then keeping that elbow back and still, bend the lower arm to the starting position. Repeat 12 times, then change legs and repeat with the other arm. Rest, then do another set of 12 with each arm.

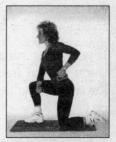

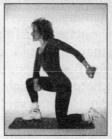

8 UPPER BACK STRENGTHENER

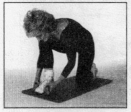

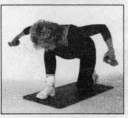

Kneel on one knee and have the front leg bent at a 90-degree angle. Rest your chest on your front knee. Holding a handweight in each hand, place your hands to either side of the front foot. Now, under control, take your bent arms out to the sides and squeeze the shoulder blades together, then lower the arms again. Repeat 6 times. Rest, then repeat.

Section Six:
Lower Body

If you are starting your workout with this section, warm up first (see page 199). After completing the lower body exercises, turn to the cool-down stretches on page 230.

1 OUTER THIGH TONER

Lie on your side, with your hips stacked and your head supported on one hand. Hold a handweight in the other hand and rest it on the outer thigh of the top leg. Bend the bottom leg at a 90-degree angle. Keeping the top leg straight, lift the leg about 20cm (8 inches), hold for a moment then lift the leg a little higher to just above hip height. Hold for a moment, then lower to the midway position, hold again for a moment, then lower the leg so that it is just off the floor. Repeat 10 times, using the handweight as resistance and without letting the leg touch the floor. Roll over and repeat with the other leg.

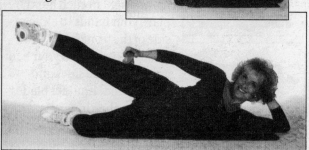

2 HIP AND OUTER THIGH TONER

Lie on your side, with your hips stacked, tummy
pulled in tight to support your back and your head
supported on one hand. Hold a handweight in the
other hand and rest it on the outer thigh of the top leg.
Bend the bottom leg at a 90-degree angle. Bend the top
leg in towards the chest, then extend it away from you
and lift it off the floor, keeping the toes pointing
forwards. Lower the leg again so that it is just off the
floor, then repeat. Repeat 10 times, using the
handweight as resistance and without letting the leg
touch the floor. Roll over and repeat with the other leg.

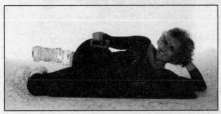

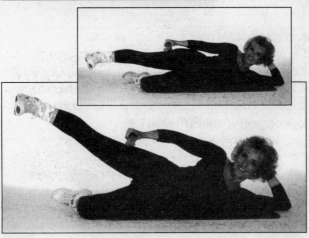

3 INNER THIGH TONER

Lie on your side, with your top leg placed behind your body as shown and foot flat on the floor. Raise the upper body onto your forearm, lifting out of your waist and pulling your tummy tight to support your back. Hold a handweight in the other hand. Straighten the

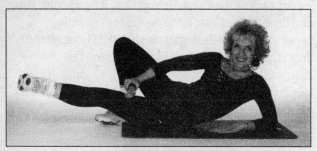

front leg and rest the hand with the handweight on the inner thigh to add resistance. Raise the leg and lower it under control. Repeat 10 times, rest, then repeat. Roll over and repeat on the other side.

4 LYING BOTTOM TONER

Lie on your front and rest your chin on your arms. Keeping your hips facing the floor, raise one leg off the floor, then lower it again and repeat with the other leg. Squeeze your bottom as you lift and lower alternate legs. Repeat 16 times (8 each leg).

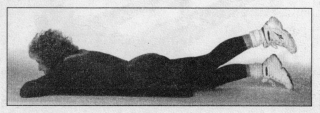

5 BOTTOM TONER

Come up onto your forearms and knees, making sure your knees are directly under your hips. Pull your tummy in tight to support your back. Extend one leg behind and rest the toes on the floor. Moving slowly and under control, lift the leg to hip height, then lower it again. Repeat, squeezing your bottom as you lift the leg and keeping your hips facing the floor. Repeat 10 times, then repeat with the other leg.

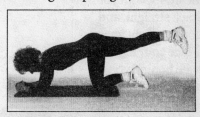

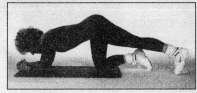

6 HAMSTRING TONER

Still resting on your forearms and knees, extend one leg behind you, level with the hip. Keeping the knee at the same height, slowly bend the leg, then straighten it again. Repeat 8 times, moving the leg slowly and under control and breathing normally throughout. Relax, then repeat with the other leg.

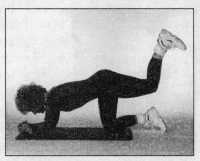

Cool-down Stretches

1 CHEST STRETCH
Sit in a comfortable cross-legged position, with your back straight, and look straight ahead. Place your hands well behind you on the floor. Ease your shoulder blades together and feel the stretch across the front of your chest. Hold for 8 seconds, then relax.

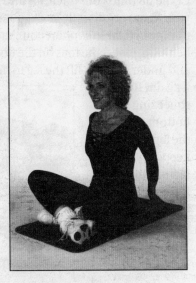

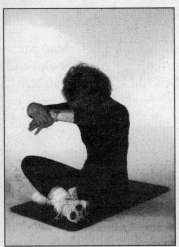

2 UPPER BACK STRETCH
Sit with your legs comfortably crossed, back straight and tummy pulled in tight. Press your arms out in front at shoulder height, lowering your head slightly, and feel the stretch in your upper back. Hold for 8 seconds, then relax.

3 OUTER THIGH AND WAIST STRETCH

Sitting upright with your legs out in front, take your left leg over your right knee and place the foot flat on the floor. Slowly twist your upper body to the left, placing your left hand behind you and using the other hand to gently ease the knee further across your body. Try to keep your

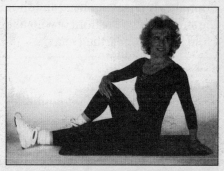

upper body upright and hold for 10 seconds. Relax, then change sides and repeat.

4 TRICEPS STRETCH

Sit in a comfortable cross-legged position, with your back straight and your head facing forwards. Bend one arm behind the shoulder and take the other arm across your chest

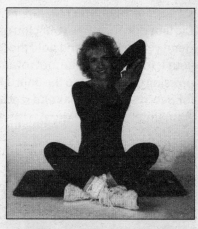

to ease the bent arm further back. Hold for 8 seconds. Relax, then repeat with the other arm.

5 TUMMY STRETCH

Lie face down on the floor. Bend your arms and position them so that the elbows are in line with the shoulders. Keeping your forearms and elbows on the floor, slowly raise your head and shoulders and feel the stretch down the front of your abdominal area. Hold for 8 seconds, then relax.

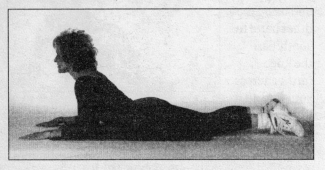

6 FRONT OF THIGH STRETCH

Lie face down, resting your chin on your right hand. Bend your left knee and hold the top of the foot with your left hand. Ease the foot towards your bottom, pressing your hips into the floor. Do not strain. Hold for 8 seconds, then relax and repeat with the other leg.

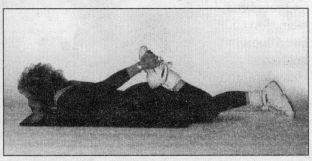

7 BOTTOM STRETCH

Lie on your back, with knees bent. Ease one knee towards your chest, placing your hands around the back of the thigh to assist. Ease the leg in as close as is comfortable and hold for 10 seconds. Relax, then repeat with the other leg.

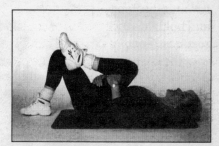

8 HAMSTRING STRETCH

Lie on your back, with knees bent. Bring one leg in towards the chest, then straighten the leg, supporting it with one hand on the back of the thigh and the other hand behind the calf. Keeping your head on the floor, ease the leg as close to your chest as possible and hold for 10 seconds. Ease the leg a little closer and hold

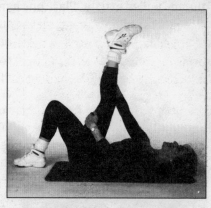

for a further 10 seconds. Bend the leg and gently lower it to the floor. Repeat with the other leg.

9 INNER THIGH STRETCH

Sit with the soles of your feet together and your elbows resting on the insides of your knees. Gently press with the elbows to ease the knees further

towards the floor and hold for 10 seconds. Now ease the knees down a little more and hold for a further 10 seconds. Relax.

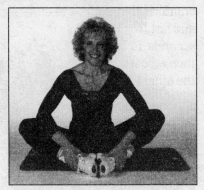

10 WAIST STRETCH

Sit with legs comfortably crossed, back straight and tummy pulled in tight. Place one hand on the floor for

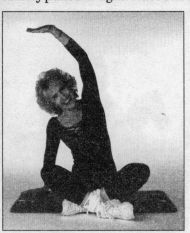

support and, lifting out of your waist, reach the other arm up towards the ceiling then over your head. Hold for 10 seconds, then relax. Repeat with the other arm.

11 SPINE STRETCH

Sit in a comfortable cross-legged position, with tummy pulled in tight. Place your hands on the floor in front of you and relax your upper body forwards, rounding your back. Breathe normally and hold for 8 seconds.

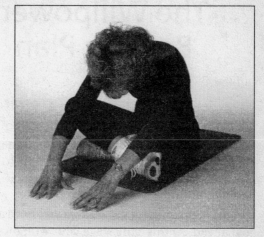

8

The Willpower
Booster Plan

Well done! The very fact that you've turned to this chapter is a really good sign. You want to succeed and have recognised the warning signs of wavering.

When you first embark on a slimming campaign you make decisions, take actions and have a definite goal ahead. At this early stage your willpower is very strong. You go shopping for all the right foods, you're dedicated in your new eating and exercise habits, you don't cheat and you can't wait for the first weigh-in at the end of the week. And the result is good. You're several pounds down, the skirt or the trousers are definitely looser, you're feeling great – and justly so.

But then three or four weeks into your campaign your rate of weight loss has slowed down. You are familiar with the diet and have become used to the menus. In fact you are perhaps too relaxed about the quantities you are eating and, if you are really honest, you'll probably find you're eating more than you should. Also ask yourself if you are doing as much exercise as you did when you started out. If you are not losing weight, you're either eating too much or doing too little – or both! But to put this into practice you need lots of willpower, so here are some tips.

Find a 'slim' photograph

Find a photograph of yourself when you were slim and keep it on display. Look at it hard and often. This is how you are going to look again *soon*, and the quicker you start towards that goal the better.

Realise that every little helps

Every day that you've been 'good' on the diet takes you a step nearer your goal. You won't see progress every day – it takes time. When a gardener sows seeds he doesn't expect to see shoots sprouting through the soil the next day. Think of your diet and fitness campaign in the same way and imagine that you are sowing seeds. When you've reached your goal, you will see that beautiful flower.

Mix with positive people

Ring a positive pal when you feel you're flagging and need a boost. He or she will encourage you, be supportive and lend a sympathetic ear. Everyone wants to feel needed, and helping a friend to become slim and healthy is a tonic to them as well as you. They will be glad to help and support you.

Weigh out what you lose

As you lose each pound off your body, place the equivalent weight (such as a tin of food, book or other object) into a carrier bag. Keep adding to the bag each week as you continue to lose weight. If you ever find yourself forgetting just how much you have achieved, just go and lift that bag and realise just how well you have done.

It is so easy for us to dismiss our progress. Having your weight bag tucked away in a cupboard or wardrobe to act as a constant reminder will provide you with a great deal of encouragement.

See the fat

Go to a butcher's and ask him for a 2.2kg (5lb) lump of fat. If you have a large deep freeze, buy the fat and freeze it. Seeing that great lump of adipose tissue is the surest way to realise what you've taken away from your body. Just think how great your body will look when you lose even more!

Clear out your wardrobes, cupboards and drawers

It is really good to have a sort out, and getting rid of all your old large clothes is really therapeutic. Save just one item – the largest garment you have – as a memento of where you have come from and how well you have done. Never part with that one.

Make a master plan

Make a list of all the things you really would love to do in life. You don't need to show it to anyone, so you can be really bold in what you write. As you get slimmer and more confident, aim to start achieving those goals. Enrol at night school for a subject you've yearned to tackle. What about driving lessons? Or perhaps you'd like to help others by doing some charity work – there's always something that needs doing, no matter what your personal circumstances may be.

Keep a success scrapbook

At Rosemary Conley Diet & Fitness Clubs, members are presented with certificates for their achievements – for being slimmer of the week, for each stone lost, and for reaching their goal. These certificates are treasured by everyone who receives them – and quite rightly so. They are tangible evidence of success.

To help you stick to your diet and fitness campaign, start keeping any scraps of evidence of your progress. This could be the gift card you received with some flowers from your partner when you lost your first stone, a letter that someone wrote to you telling you how well and trim you looked, the date your doctor confirmed your blood pressure went down. Write down any verbal compliments you receive. Stick in photographs of yourself taken as you lose each stone. Jot down the date you bought a smaller size skirt and how you felt – anything that is positive. Then on those bad days when your willpower is flagging, just glance through your scrapbook and give yourself a boost. At such times, reading kind comments made about us can lift our spirits and make us realise that our efforts are paying dividends after all.

Celebrate

For each stone you lose celebrate with a special occasion – a meal out with friends, a trip to the theatre, a day at a health spa. Plan to do something that is really exciting and that will spur you on to even greater success. It is good to reward ourselves when we have achieved a goal – it builds confidence and makes each goal special.

9

Maintaining Your New Body

It's often said that losing weight is relatively easy and that keeping it off is the difficult part. To some degree this is an oversimplified statement as, for many people, losing weight takes a huge amount of will-power and commitment. We are faced with temptation at every corner and only the most dedicated will arrive at that goal. However, maintaining your new weight really can be simpler than you might think.

During one of my recording sessions for Granada Sky Broadcasting (GSB) I was talking to Dr Andrew Prentice from the Dunn Nutrition Centre. We were discussing the likelihood of people regaining weight after losing it on a weight-reducing diet and Dr Prentice told a very interesting story about a weight-control trial conducted with Boston policemen.

These rather weighty Americans were all given a weight-reducing diet and an exercise regime to follow over a period of weeks. They all lost weight and no doubt felt significantly better for it. Next, they were divided into two groups. The first group was told that they had finished the trial and they could carry on in whatever way they wished. The second group was told that they had finished the weight-reducing diet but were asked to continue with the exercise programme. Interestingly, the members of the first group regained all their weight after several months, whereas the members of the second group, who continued to exercise, kept their lost weight off.

There is conclusive evidence that those people who exercise regularly stand a far better chance of maintaining a trim figure. This is why I can't emphasise enough the importance of continuing to exercise regularly once you have reached your goal weight. Make it a part of your lifestyle. Join a sports club, go to a gym or an exercise class, or work out to a fitness video with a friend. Enter your exercise sessions into your diary and make sure you stick to them. Exercise should become a habit, and the longer you keep up those sports and fitness habits, the more they will become entrenched into your lifestyle and the greater the chance you will have of maintaining your new figure.

As far as food is concerned, the rules are equally simple. Once you have reached your goal weight, you may gradually increase the amount of food you eat, but I would still emphasise the importance of eating low fat. You can increase the fat threshold from four to five per cent when selecting goods from the supermarket shelves. This will extend the variety of foods that you can choose and give you greater freedom.

I recommend you still stick to your three-main-meals-a-day routine. You can, of course, include snacks similar to the ones included in the New Body Diet, although I strongly suggest that you avoid getting into the habit of grazing between meals, as it's so easy to consume more calories than you realise. If at any point in the future you find your weight creeping up by a pound or two, then just cut back on the quantities or return to the diet. It will only take a few days to regulate your weight and the sooner it is done the better.

Make it a rule not to weigh yourself more than once a week and make sure you weigh yourself on the same scales at the same time of day each week, wearing the same clothes or preferably none. Try to become more confident and develop the sense of feeling in control of your food intake rather than letting it control you. The last thing you want to do is become obsessed about what you are eating.

The good news is that when dining out or attending a special celebration you can feel free to eat what you like and enjoy it. The occasional indulgence won't do any harm and should be greatly appreciated. Having the odd slice of gateau or serving of chips is not the greatest sin in the world. Enjoy it, but just don't have it every day!

If at all possible, when you reach your goal weight, treat yourself to some new outfits. A new wardrobe of clothes is a powerful incentive to keeping you slim. When you see how wonderful you look in your fabulous new clothes, you will never want to go back to your old habits or your old large sizes.

Learn to accept compliments. If someone tells you that you look lovely and slim, then accept it as you would accept a gift. Saying 'I worked really hard but I feel great and ten years younger' is a much better response than 'Oh, I've still got a big tummy/thighs/backside ...' If somebody pays you a compliment, it's because they feel it's warranted. So make them feel glad that they said it. You will probably be getting a lot more as the weeks and months go on so it's worth perfecting the art of accepting them.

Index of Recipes

Goal Chart

Start weight .... Start date	Goal weight .... Target date	Motivating reason (e.g. treat, wedding, dinner & dance etc.)
1st target .... Lose ....lb By .... (date)	Actual weight loss........ Inches lost to date........ Date........	
2nd target .... Lose ....lb By .... (date)	Actual weight loss........ Inches lost to date........ Date........	
3rd target .... Lose ....lb By .... (date)	Actual weight loss........ Inches lost to date........ Date........	

	4th target_____ Lose_____lb By_____(date)	Actual weight loss_____ Inches lost to date_____ Date_____
	5th target_____ Lose_____lb By_____(date)	Actual weight loss_____ Inches lost to date_____ Date_____
	6th target_____ Lose_____lb By_____(date)	Actual weight loss_____ Inches lost to date_____ Date_____
	Final target_____ Lose_____lb By_____(date)	Actual weight loss_____ Inches lost to date_____ Date_____

Measurement Record Chart

DATE	WEIGHT	BUST	WAIST	HIPS	WIDEST PART

MEASUREMENT RECORD CHART

TOP OF THIGHS		ABOVE KNEES		UPPER ARMS		COMMENTS
L	R	L	R	L	R	

Weight-loss Graph

Make up your own graph for each stone you lose, following the example below.

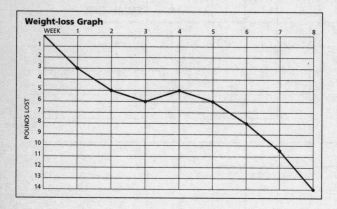

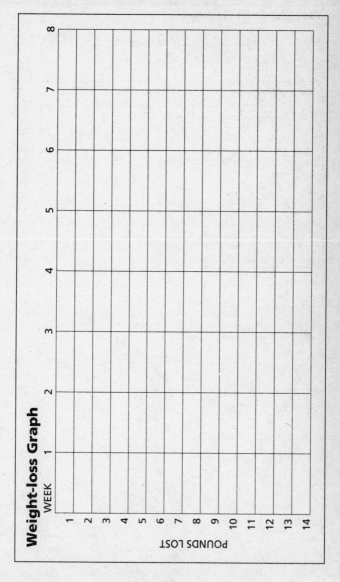

Weight-loss Graph

WEEK

POUNDS LOST

NEW BODY
by
Design

Work out in the comfort of your own home with Rosemary Conley's New Body By Design video, which forms the ideal complement to this book.

Reshape your body as never before with this fabulous workout video that combines low-impact aerobics with controlled upper body conditioning in the same moves, resulting in a very safe and time-effective workout. Suitable for all levels of fitness, the video allows you to design your own exercise regime. It contains six ten-minute routines, each of which targets a specific area of the body – hips and thighs, upper arms, chest and upper back, abdominals and back, upper body, lower body – so that you can concentrate on your particular problem area.

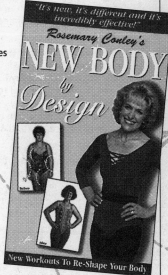

Rosemary Conley's New Body By Design video is published by VCI, priced at £10.99, and is available from all good retail video stockists.

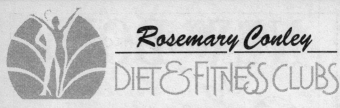

Rosemary Conley

DIET & FITNESS CLUBS

FRANCHISE OPPORTUNITY

We are looking for quality people to expand our network of franchises across the United Kingdom. All franchisees are personally selected by Rosemary Conley and receive full training which includes, if necessary, the RSA basic Certificate in Exercise to Music qualification.

Franchisees follow an established formula with professional backup and ongoing training. Our aim is for our franchisees' businesses to be highly successful. If you are interested in a franchise with Rosemary Conley Diet and Fitness Clubs, please ask yourself the following questions:

1 Are you prepared to benefit from the Company's extensive training programme?
2 Operating a Rosemary Conley Diet and Fitness franchise is a full-time career. Are you prepared to give up your present employment?
3 Do you regularly participate in exercise classes?
4 Are you aged between 23 and 45 years?

If you have answered 'yes' to all of these questions and would like to receive more information about this exciting business opportunity, please complete the form below and return it to:

Rosemary Conley Diet and Fitness Clubs Ltd
Ref: NBP/1, Quorn House, Meeting Street,
Quorn, Loughborough,
Leicestershire, LE12 8EX

Alternatively telephone (01509) 620222 and ask for a Prospectus.

- -

Please send me a Prospectus on the Rosemary Conley Diet and Fitness Clubs Franchise.

Name: _____

Address: _____

_____

Age: _____   Are you RSA qualified? _____

Rosemary Conley

DIET & FITNESS CLUBS

Rosemary Conley Diet and Fitness Clubs help you to achieve a slimmer, fitter and healthier lifestyle. You can follow Rosemary Conley's diet in the company of others and benefit from weekly exercise, encouragement, advice and support.

Every class offers a weigh-in, presentation of a certificate to the 'Slimmer of the Week', followed by a 45-minute workout taught by a qualified instructor.

The classes are suitable for all fitness levels and, whether you have a little or a lot to lose, our specially trained instructors will ensure you are made very welcome. You will receive all the help and encouragement that you need with the diet and the exercises.

All franchisees are personally selected by Rosemary Conley and are trained to achieve the Royal Society of Arts Exercise to Music qualification in association with the Sports Council, and have also attended the Rosemary Conley Diet and Fitness Club Training Course.

**For details of classes in your area call
01509 620222**

At Last –

**A DIET AND FITNESS CLUB THAT COMBINES
A HEALTHY LOW-FAT DIET WITH SAFE AND
EFFECTIVE EXERCISE CLASSES**

Rosemary Conley

DIET & FITNESS

MAGAZINE

Save up to £10 on standard subscription rates!

Enjoy new diet ideas, exercises and recipes, plus amazing success stories, celebrity interviews, competitions and giveaways. Each issue, out every other month, will be sent direct to you post-free and ahead of the on-sale date.

Subscribe now for the next six issues and we'll send you a FREE Rosemary Conley Diet & Fitness T-shirt worth £5 OR enjoy the next 12 issues and receive the Rosemary Conley Diet & Fitness Record Book worth £3.99, plus the T-shirt – all absolutely FREE. The book allows you to record your meals, exercise, weekly weight and inch loss as well as being a pocket reference for fat content values, exercise and includes Rosemary's diet tips.

Simply phone the **Credit Card Hotline 01858 435363** or complete and return the form below, enclosing your cheque or postal order.

SUBSCRIPTION ORDER FORM

FREE GIFTS

YES, I would like to subscribe for:

☐ 12 issues – £20 (FREE T-SHIRT and

Diet & Fitness Record Book) (003)

☐ 6 issues – £10 (FREE T-SHIRT) (002)

I enclose cheque/PO for £_____ , payable to Quorn House Publishing Ltd.

Mr/Mrs/Miss/Ms _____

Address _____

_____

Postcode _____ Telephone _____

**Rosemary Conley Diet & Fitness Magazine,
FREEPOST (LE6740), Market Harborough, LE87 4DZ**

Offer closes 31 December 1997, gifts available while stocks last.

Rosemary Conley Diet & Fitness Magazine offers you the opportunity to receive information from respected organisations about their products and services. Please tick if you prefer not to receive these ☐

0010